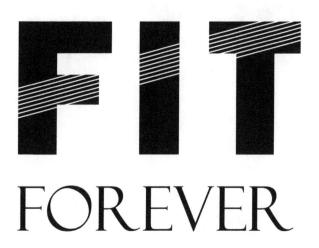

FIT
FOREVER

Amber Dobecka

ISBN 979-8-89043-704-4 (paperback)
ISBN 979-8-89043-705-1 (digital)

Christian Faith Publishing
832 Park Avenue
Meadville, PA 16335
www.christianfaithpublishing.com

Printed in the United States of America

To Yahweh, my Lord God, to whom I seek to serve and worship through this book.

To my forever love, the best friend I ever had, the father of my children, and my partner in the journey, Micah, without whom I'd still be lost in the woods. Thank you for choosing to look at me through rose-colored glasses. You've been the most obvious means of God's grace, love, and faithfulness in my life.

And to my kids, Lincoln, Titus, and Sunny. You have taught me more than you'll ever know.

CONTENTS

    This is an explanation of why spiritual transformation trumps physical transformation and how your purpose and potential are revealed in the rhythm of pursuing God through discipline and grace. This is an overview of why progress is more important than perfection and how that relates to both physical and spiritual wellness.

    This chapter reveals the most underemphasized character trait and the importance of how we position ourselves in relation to God and others. Stories of humility and humiliation provide a practical look at how our position can place us on the path toward purpose.

    Discovering our disappointments and dysfunction serves as an opportunity to get stronger from the inside out. This chapter shares raw accounts of pain to demonstrate how heartache can lead to heart change.

Information is not enough; we must understand how the application of knowledge through discipline is key to consistent growth in every area of our life. A list of spiritual disciplines and how to practically pursue God through discipline is included.

This chapter teaches you how to apply discipline to your physical wellness and why it's important. It also includes practical tips to alter habits of nutrition and exercise.

This chapter teaches you how to apply discipline to your mental wellness and why it's important. It includes practical ways to reflect on how to identify lies you've believed and replace them with godly truth in your thoughts.

This chapter teaches you how to apply discipline to your emotional wellness and why it's important. It includes how to practice self-awareness and self-control to harness the power of God-given emotions.

This chapter gives you an understanding that moving from motivation to discipline requires character development. The choices we make in times of struggle are the ones that make us stronger.

Identifying what builds our faith and how to get more of it is imperative to being spiritually fit. This chapter explains how strengthening oneself requires redirecting our thoughts, feeling, and actions to biblical roots.

Learning how to set your soul up even when you're
unhappy is one of the hardest mental workouts, but doing
so will keep you on the journey toward spiritual fitness.

This is the driving force that keeps our rhythm on pace
with exercising our God-given purpose and fulfilling our
potential. It's this part of the process of spiritual wellness
that reenergizes our efforts to keep getting stronger from
the inside out.

Here is a final call to action to apply the knowledge learned
from my journey to starting yours. Becoming fit forever is
a process, one that must be inspired and shared.

INTRODUCTION

THIS BOOK WAS *going* to be a sexy spin on spiritual fitness.

This book was *going* to be for anyone who was frustrated with their weight or body image.

This book was *going* to be adorned with trendy, low-carb recipes and DIY home workouts.

This book was *going* to be a book for people who had unsuccessfully dieted or lacked the keys to physical confidence, which I thought I would include.

This book was *going* to be much like many other books whose pages promise they will help you figure out why you feel the way you do and what you need to do to fix it.

And then this book just didn't get written. For years, I delayed writing this book—no book at all! And by the time I finally felt like I couldn't put it off any longer, my reasons for writing the dang book changed all together. My life took turn after turn, setting me on a course that ironically led me to a much more profound purpose than writing anything at all.

Everything about my life has changed. At least, it seems that way. On the surface, there are only a few things that have changed, but I think that's the point. Most of the transformation has taken place way down deep, within the foundations of my soul. It's the idea of soul transformation that originally intrigued me about writing a book that was unlike others in the first place. It's what kept me disappointed in life for a long time. The presence of this longing in my soul to find purpose beyond checking off goals and attaining success is what kept me pursuing self-improvement. Because the thought of improving myself gave me hope that my contentment in life would improve too. At first, I sought improvement in my glutes, waist, and mile time. Now I see that was just the setup for total soul transformation.

The first time I remember having a serious thought about capturing my ideas in a book, I was a professional fitness instructor. I use the term *professional* because the fitness industry is filled with all kinds of exercise gurus, and that was one thing I wanted to esteem: that I was a professional.

Before I turned thirty years old, I had ten years of experience and folders filled with certifications. This is relevant because the fitness industry has influenced so much of my mindset. It has helped me understand the importance of discipline and self-control in concrete ways. I lived and breathed wellness, and I loved helping others.

As I sought my own wellness, I learned that aesthetic goals were attractive, but holistic wellness was where it was at. Years of sweating and training and kicking butts (including my own) taught me that if I was going to keep this up, I'd need to find something beyond a better body image to keep me from burnout.

Exercise and the pursuit of wellness really and truly helped me along in my relationship with God. The collision of physical fitness and spiritual fitness eventually brought me to a place where I felt disconnected from the fitness industry all together. Still, I fought to keep myself successful as a trainer and instructor. It was as if I thought that the longer I trained my body to persevere past pain, the stronger my soul would get. What I didn't understand is that my soul actually didn't need to get stronger. It needed to die.

It's all about me.

Death of one's soul is not a theme prevalent among former fitness instructors. It's actually quite contradictory. For years, I fought myself over how to approach my job as a coach, trainer, and aspiring fitness model. I was in an industry that dotes on "You can, and you will. You're enough." Yet I felt like the truth that kept knocking at my door was saying, "No, you actually can't. You're not enough." The collision of these opposing messages created internal conflict.

Although on the surface, the attitude of the latter statement seems negative and possibly degrading, what I found in God's Word was that it actually was more truthful than the first. Without the spirit of Christ consuming every part of my soul, I *can't* do it. I *won't* do it. And I'm *not* enough. This totally contradicts not only the fitness industry but also the basic fibers of American society. And that's why I decided that my original intent to share my story without weaving the gospel within every line was plumb dumb.

My fitness career began as a hobby, but the emphasis on exercise began when I was a kid. Memories of my mom's jazzercise and step classes appear throughout my adolescence. Accompanied by memories of self-hatred, punishment, and exercise addiction, fitness has been a major theme in my life for as long as I can remember. To combat the lies of the enemy, which sounded a lot like the words from others, I tried to train my body to be as beautiful, fit, and strong as I thought I should be—to become as perfect as I thought I could be.

Working out and watching what I ate was just one way I found purpose in performing for others. I was determined to excel in every area of which I could control. This meant I considered myself a failure unless I seemingly maintained perfection. In school, it meant a perfect GPA and early graduation. At my childhood home, it meant mothering my three young brothers and counseling my parents' marriage. Professionally, it meant becoming a sought-after trainer and fitness model. Later in my own marriage, it meant proactively meeting all my husbands' needs. And much later in motherhood, it meant maintaining well-behaved children who would rise up and call me *blessed*. While I thought I was selflessly giving to others, I was both tolerating the taking and trying to control everyone else around me.

If God's not at the center of everything you do, then something's out of place. I realized I'd placed myself at the center of every relationship and every endeavor so that everything affected me.

Today, I can see how the enemy uses every God-given gift as a trap to keep me focused on myself. This doesn't mean I'm not allowed to have seasons where I'm struggling and seeking healing and freedom. But the latter part of that idea must exist. What does it mean to seek healing and freedom? Does the number of followers I have indicate I'm healthy and free? Does the number of likes I have indicate my worth? Does the weight of my career or lack thereof indicate my purpose? Is self-care really as important as it seems among empowering social groups? Do my feelings even matter, or should I totally disregard how I feel? And if so, what does that look like through God's eyes?

These are questions I've pondered for years. If I want the truth, then I must go to the author of truth. I must seek answers that are beyond social media screenshots and self-making seminars.

It's not about me.

All of us are navigating life in a system that glorifies self. If we're not intentional at glorifying God, we probably will fall right along in that system. That's where I was, and that's where I still occasionally find myself. Even when I'm off social media, I tend to find myself viewing my husband and my kids as extensions of myself. For years, I held my husband accountable to the standard I had for myself. For years, I routinely gave into feelings of guilt, disappointment, shame, doubt, and fear. I didn't yet understand that God was calling me to break free from the standard I had made for myself and indirectly reflected on others.

So does this mean I no longer workout or watch what I eat? Absolutely not! Like I mentioned before, some of what I was doing wasn't really wrong; it was *why* I was doing them that was so wrong. Undoubtedly, God speaks to me when I'm active, whether I'm pushing my kids in the jogging stroller, or I've got headphones on, and the world turned off. But the reality is that much of what God wanted me to learn has to do with the dying of self instead of the improvement of self.

So why write another book about knowing yourself and knowing God?

To inspire people.

Inspired people change the world even when they feel frustrated, discouraged, and unnoticed. Inspired people move past the motivated because their actions don't solely rely on emotion, but they're also driven by discipline. God calls us to discipline when He commands our obedience. He commands it out of His sovereignty, but He also desires our yielded will. He wants us to enjoy life to our fullest potential.

> Those whom I love, I reprove and discipline, so
> be zealous and repent. (Revelation 3:19 ESV)

As our creator, He knows what we're capable of, and He knows why we exist. Although people have been exploring the question of our life's purpose for years, I think we humans are still missing it as a whole. If we weren't, this book and others like it would be irrelevant. In an age where technology, information, and social structures are at their peak, we still find ourselves lost in isolation and futility. We're still surrounded by fake love, false humility, and foolish independence. We still see people suffer without hope. We still see people hurt themselves. We still see the world desperate to cling to some form of unified truth and inspiration.

> Writing is the only way I have to explain my own
> life to myself. (Pat Conroy, *My Reading Life*)

This is why I need to be inspired.

This book is merely a compilation of journal entries, middle-of-the-night notes, and reflections on seeking God in the presence of pain. Now that I'm officially writing it, I see how this is an exercise to inspire *me* just as much as it is to inspire someone else. I mean that not in a conceited way but in the most humble way I know how to express.

I need inspiration—daily—sometimes, every five minutes, whether I'm cleaning up another sticky mess from one of my toddlers or losing it in an epic breakdown behind the scenes. I struggle. We all do if we're honest. Recording the faithful whisper of the Father in how He has spoken to me personally and corporately and sharing the insight gleaned from these gut-wrenching moments inspires me.

This is why others need to be inspired.

There's also reason to believe people need to be inspired as I've observed societal transformation. People are desperately seeking validation. I know I was. It's apparent all over social media. It's obvious as more and more stories of suicide, depression, and division are making headlines.

Today, people value their voice and want to be heard, to the point our world has accepted that each person should have the right to live *their own truth*. The problem is that there cannot be various forms of truth. It simply contradicts the definition of truth. People need to hear and see and experience the real truth, even if they don't know it yet.

> Whoever loves discipline loves knowledge, but he
> who hates reproof is stupid. (Proverbs 12:1 ESV)

If knowledge is power, then truth is undeniably life-changing. I think we have a fair share of knowledge available to people; it's truth we're missing. But like Theodore Roosevelt said, "People don't care how much you know until they know how much you care." There's no more effective way at spreading God's truth than sharing how it's been applicable to my own story. When others hear (or read) that someone else is relatable, they can use that example and apply the principles to their own situation, thus becoming better at inspiring others.

So what do I mean when I talk about being inspired?

> All scripture is God-breathed [given by divine inspiration] and is profitable for instruction, for conviction [of sin], for correction [of error and restoration to obedience], for training in righteousness [learning to live in conformity to God's will, both publicly and privately—behaving honorably with personal integrity and moral courage]. (2 Timothy 3:16 AMP)

Divine inspiration. Those words literally mean God breathed out to create all things and formulate thoughts that would translate to words on a page—the Bible. And since we're created in His image, we can inspire as well. To be inspired means to be moved from the inside out. When you're inspired, you're driven by something internally bigger than yourself.

I'll address this in much more detail later, but this contradicts a similar word. When I refer to being motivated, I mean being moved by an outside force. When you're motivated, you're driven by something external, and it usually causes you to desire some sort of external change like appearance, behavior, or status. In my experience, motivation works temporarily. Inspiration can have lasting momentum. I conclude I need inspiration when I find that my feelings are outweighing my desire. Many times, my motivation runs out when other people's motivation wears out too. Inspiration is evident when I keep doing the right things and keep persevering even when I'm by myself.

Even in writing this book, I had to ask myself the hard questions that revealed how much of my desire was tied to external forces. That's why it took me years to get brave enough to start intentionally writing and editing.

So as I sit here today, I can honestly tell you, that it's in desperation that I found inspiration. It wasn't scrolling through Instagram and seeing a bunch of influencers' posts that made me go, "Oh yes, that's what I'll do." In fact, I've had to stay off social media all together for over a year before being able to start writing. In doing so, I began to feel disconnected and unseen. I've battled thoughts of worthlessness and brokenness that drove me to make a decision.

Was I going to keep blowing the party pipe at my own pity party, or was I going to confess to God and call out for His voice?

Hearing His voice awoke my own.

As I share my story (and I will along the way), I inspire myself. I'm reiterating to my soul the power of God's truth. I can look back at how I've struggled and how I'm still standing and more importantly *why*. That reflection is best done in the community so that my story has a chance at helping someone else clarify their own. It's not that my story is any different or worse than many others, but it's the fact that every story matters to God. My intention is to be real with you, dear friend. There are enough filtered highlight reels of people we want to be like out there already. So if you're expecting to read how I have it all together, you should quit reading now.

To truly inspire myself and others, I must commit to the truth. And the reality is that I've only discovered more and more of God's truth from one mistake after another—from abuse to unfaithfulness to a whole new me. If I don't share how my suffering makes me stronger, then I may be missing an opportunity to inspire someone else. The insight I hope to reveal may equip others to have a perspective change on what being strong means according to God and what it means to know God and, therefore, know yourself, and to understand how dependence on God alone gets us there.

You were created to inspire.

Being inspirational is more than a catchy meme. It's more than a phrase spoken over a microphone to a room of indoor cyclists. It's loving on purpose; it's creating a theme for your life that reflects one's intention and making sure that theme is apparent throughout the thread work of your life. And in this context, it means to shine God's light.

If you can catch how I struggle to implement a habit of discipline in all areas of my life, you will feel validated in your own weakness. If you also gain some understanding of God's epic love, to which I will boast, then maybe you'll begin to depend on His love instead of other forms of validation. So much of this wisdom I've learned from patterns of disobedience and the consequences that follow.

Like any good person would do, if I can share with you what I've learned, both sparing suffering and sparking perspective change, then I will. Sharing how the application of discipline has transformed my relationship with God and all other relationships is key. And more than just inspiration, I hope to offer you practical applications to improving godly habits in all areas of your life and demonstrate how this insight has brought freedom, healing, and peace to my own.

So when you're ready, flip the page. Jump into the journey ahead. Pray alongside me and ask what God wants to speak to you through the pages of this story.

CHAPTER 1

THE JOURNEY

AWAKE BUT LIFELESS in my soul, I lay in my empty bed, thinking about what I'd tell my boss to explain why I wasn't at work yet. Quickly, as if the speed at which I typed out my email would help ease the guilt of lying again, I hit "Send."

I wasn't stuck in traffic. I was stuck in my grief. My guilt. My shame. Hopelessness consumed my emotions as I realized the gravity of my consistent failure at being a good wife. Mistakes were made. Sin separated me from my husband. The weight of my discontent crushed me. Many mornings, like this one, I found myself in the fetal position. The sheets over my face didn't hide me enough. I wanted to be hidden away from everyone and everything. *I deserved to die*, I thought. *I deserved nothing and owed everything.* This was a lie from the enemy, but it was mixed with a little truth, proven by my past and my feelings.

I don't remember how or when, but I know I eventually got out of bed that day. I managed to function with the shame and the guilt and this hole in my heart. As the days passed, and the desperation swelled in my soul, I realized that hole had always been there; I'd just never acknowledged it before. I'd filled it with prideful attempts to achieve perfection and convinced myself that I could control myself and others enough to arrive at happiness.

1

Blatantly sinful choices exposed my inherent nature. I was no better than anyone. Had I thought I was? Had I thought that I was better, more righteous, than others? Had I thought that sin was beyond me? I'd never admitted those beliefs, but my actions revealed otherwise. I found myself in this season facing a part of myself I'd never seen, almost as if I was living a double life.

The Bible says, "A double-minded man is unstable in all his ways" (James 1:8). Oh yeah, I was unstable alright. Yet I'd always believed myself to be so sure of my values, my principles, my confidence...in myself. That was the open door. Believing in myself and relying on my own power to handle life led me to a place where I saw how epically flawed I was. I'm thankful for the revelation. I owe it to God pursuing me even while I fled Him. I owe it to prayers over me from a young age and the doors opened to His presence early on in my life. I owe it to the faith and grace operative in my loved ones, especially my husband.

While my husband, Micah, might share a different view on this season of our life, from my perspective, he was the earthly demonstration of God's love in action to me. I can look back and truly testify to my own growth by remembering my husband's godly actions and extension of grace to me. I can look back without harboring any offense at how he may have also hurt me because, through my husband, God could heal me.

That's what people do though. We hurt each other. And that's how evil infects us—by allowing the offenses to inflame so that we never totally heal or totally forgive. Instead, we either create walls, or we heal and partially forgive. And finally, we continue the cycle of blaming and shaming.

This is what I'm free of now. And this is why I feel compelled to share my testimony as well as peel back the layers of my journey.

So many people, even those closest to me, probably see only certain layers of who I am. It's natural for us all to conclude what we think of someone based on what we see or experience. While I've never been one who could hide myself, I found myself still hidden, still operating apart from the genuine person God created me to be.

Discovering who God says I am has inspired me to say whatever I can say and to share whatever I can share so that others are drawn closer to God. Through the unveiling of our weaknesses, we discover who we truly are. Like me, we all face our flaws. Some hide them on purpose, and some don't know what's in their way until it's thrown in their face.

All of us journey, but not all of us journey forward.

> Let your eyes look directly forward, and your gaze be straight before you. (Proverbs 4:25)

As I've fallen and gotten back up, I've refocused on God. I do this daily now, not just in the big collapses but the daily frustrations of life. I've learned the only way to truly move forward is to do so with intention, with effort, and with the power of the Holy Spirit living and breathing in me.

I look back at myself and also look around at others, and I see many who are journeying through life but staying the same. I think it was a taste of this knowledge, the distaste, rather, for complacency that had me so disappointed in my life years ago, that drove me to despair. You see, I felt the lack in my life, the crusty wearing of staying the same and seeking the same, without the centered gaze upon my Creator. Time does march on, but as spiritual beings in human bodies, we're not designed to merely age and mature in earthly form. We're created to develop spiritually and holistically.

> I press on toward the goal for the prize of the upward call of God in Christ Jesus. (Philippians 3:14)

The upward call is hard work. I believe that's why there are tons of books and resources on self-development, personal growth, and success. I have no issues with these resources and have found them instrumental in my own journey forward. My hope is to include elements of spiritual growth and a testament to its power by sharing the words on these pages. However, none of those words would matter without simultaneously declaring the source of my soul transformation. All those years ago, after I decided to submit my entire soul to God, I became aware of my people-focused perspective.

When I started trying to focus on God at the center of my life, I realized how attached I was to people. I felt like I was being unloving at times. I felt alone at times. I felt many emotions and had many thoughts, yet I felt obedient to the personal voice of God for the first time ever. I'd usually not ever had a problem following the rules, but this was not that kind of obedience. This was personal and real.

The thing about the journey is that it rarely includes a 180-degree direction change. And it didn't for me either. The journey, of which I'm still on, was a slow-moving marathon with benchmarks of wisdom gleaned from desperation. If I look back, I can see a drastic directional change from where I was, but as I've journeyed, it's felt far more gradual.

Our life experiences shape who we are, but we're still in control of who we're becoming. In every season, there are both highs and lows; there are devastating setbacks and undeserving blessings. Life is full of circumstances that we cannot control. I think many like me probably get caught up trying to change things that in their power they will never be able to change, instead of changing what they can.

In my journey so far, I can see evidence of God's design in the opportunities He's given me to learn and grow. I've learned the value of discipline through exercise and my career as a wellness coach. I've learned how to practice faithfulness and trust through a long stretch of unanswered prayers. I've learned the difference between joy and happiness as I've faced one disappointment after another. I've learned how to be alone and not isolated. And I've learned of the depths of God's heart through reflection, grief, and healing.

These lessons were personal, but they were not exclusive. God has a plan for each one of His children. He desires to speak to each one personally. I've learned from having my own children that every kid is growing and requires my grace daily. This has helped me apply this truth to my own journey as a child walking beside my heavenly Father.

I'm to look forward, to move forward. I'm to heal and gain freedom from my past, to be thankful for my present, and to push toward the plans ahead. We can get so comfortable in our daily routines, our habits, and our mindsets. We can complain about things that bother us without really doing anything to change. To me, that's the most frustrating thing I can do. And yet I still do it sometimes.

> Remember not the former things, nor consider
> the things of old. (Isaiah 43:18)

Part of moving forward is forgiving myself and choosing to see myself through God's eyes. My view of how God sees me has drastically changed over the years. That's one of the messages I hope this book conveys—a more honest depiction of God's loving perspective on His children, on you.

To understand God's perspective on us, we have to know God. We have to pursue Him. We have to change from thinking about Him in dysfunctional, distorted ways. Then we have to change the way we see ourselves. With correct vision, we can both give to God and receive from Him. I've found that this exchange is what has helped me grow and helped me journey through every challenge, leaving behind the baggage of my sins and stepping into the gracious embrace of His rhythm.

Every day, I have to recall the truth: God does not see me for who I am at this moment. In His infinite wisdom, He knows everything about me, everything I've done, and everything I will do, both good and bad. His view defies the limits of time and humanity. He knows my potential and is constantly wooing me toward it. When I focus on God, every other distraction blurs out. With His help, purpose in life is clear. Even amid tragedy or heartbreaks, we can journey through life with joy, peace, and hope.

**Your purpose and potential are revealed
in the rhythm of pursuing God.**

My journey thus far has brought me to the message of this book. The call to action is clear. God wants me to put pen to paper (or finger to keyboard, rather). Even in writing this very paragraph, I wonder how God will use my words. In my flesh, I still flounder over how my story could truly help anyone else. But I have to practice what I preach and trust God.

One of the most basic messages I feel compelled to share is that your purpose and potential are revealed in the rhythm of pursuing God. I've learned there's a chain of godly character traits that propels me to sustain a purposeful livelihood. I call it a chain because I've often found that if I can start at the top, and focus on one, then it leads me to the next. It's a flow that naturally occurs when I decide to follow God.

**Humility leads me to obedience. Obedience leads me to
discipline. Discipline is the practice of faith. Practicing
faithfulness fills me with hope. Hope in my heart
brings me joy. A joyful person is a strong person.**

In other words, when I'm humble (really, truly humble, not #humblebragging), then I understand why God calls me to obey Him, which leads me to apply discipline so that I can sustain submission to Him, which teaches me how to practice faithfulness, which helps me believe God at His Word and know His thoughts toward me are ones of joy, which renews my focus on God and why He has me here on earth and how there's eternal life beyond this one, which reveals how strong I can be if I depend on God instead of myself. (Thank you for enduring the world's longest run-on sentence.)

Do I get sidetracked? Yes. Do I take the wrong turns? Yes. Do I go when I should stop? Yes. Do I stop when I should go? Yes. The pace is personal, and my prayer is that the Holy Spirit would reveal His personal plan to each person who takes the time to read this book. I've also included as many personal details as the Lord would have me share because I know that our world is desperate for authentic connection. I also trust that every painful secret shared is one the enemy loses power over in my own life. And I hope it inspires you to keep journeying forward, to not stay complacent any longer, and to, instead, take the leap and trust God one step at a time.

My words throughout the next several chapters dive headfirst into this rhythm, this pace of life. It's at this pace I've learned to journey forward.

CHAPTER 2

HUMILITY

The beginning of all discipline: humility

> And He said to all, "If anyone would come after me, let him deny himself and take up his cross daily and follow me." (Luke 9:23 ESV)

WHILE THE WORLD boasts of self-discipline, self-worth, and self-made celebrities, God says "Deny oneself." What does this really mean?

To me, this is the first place we must head. Any question of our faith or hardship we face comes back to this: humility. And yet it's the one ingredient missing in today's worldly recipe of self-love.

> Whoever exalts himself will be humbled, and whoever humbles himself will be exalted. (Matthew 23:12 ESV)

Today, we're encouraged to take pride in who we are, what we do, what we think, who we like or dislike, what we agree with, and who we designate as our tribe. Many times, this messaging is sneaky and sounds like humility or love. True humility and true love focus on God. They remove the spotlight from ourselves. It's not degrading or devaluing oneself, but it's increasing value on God. It's not defaming us, but it's esteeming God. If we're clear on what constitutes the glorification of God versus what glorifies ourselves, we can usually determine whether or not humility is present.

> When pride comes, then comes disgrace, but
> with the humble is wisdom. (Proverbs 11:2 ESV)

It's our humility that postures us as Christians to receive God's power. When we humbly admit we need Jesus, we welcome His spirit to invade our own and transform our souls to be more like His. The problem arises when we realize this transformation is a process. I believe that our belief in Christ instantly and assuredly saves my soul and gets me a ticket to spend eternity in Heaven, but it doesn't save me from suffering on earth. As I've spiritually matured and grown more and more fervent in my obsession with Jesus, it's only been through humility. It's only happened because I've tried countless times to control circumstances myself and failed.

Humility in motherhood

If you're not a momma, please bear with me, as I think there are nuggets here worth reading, even if it means using your imagination for a bit. There are few things more humbling than motherhood. The very process of becoming a momma physiologically is a lesson in humility.

For ten months (those who say nine must have never been pregnant), a woman's body is sieged, as if her very insides are being sucked out and replaced by a very self-focused being, whose intentions are to secure the body for themselves. Side effects of pregnancy can include the traditional morning sickness, fatigue, incessant urination, and less-commonly-talked-about-things like hormonal imbalances, memory loss, and the never-ever-ever-the-same postpartum *mom bod*. There are even more less-discussed side effects including excessive appearance of skin tags, hot flashes, unexplained breathlessness, and varicose veins. I know because as I wrote this, I was pregnant with my third child. Just getting up to check on my kids gets me out of breath!

I say all this humorously, although I'm well-convinced this process is no doubt miraculous—a gift—and yet most moms would agree it doesn't feel much like a gift as it's happening.

And then even the most serene pregnancies inevitably end with some sort of struggle to deliver the baby. Knees wide open and more faces as close to your downstairs as they'll ever be, a momma finds herself in the most vulnerable position thus far. Internally conflicted, she desperately wants to be told what to do, yet she also wants to scream at everyone who dares to open their mouth. The pain is unthinkable, and the show is humiliating, and yet in a matter of seconds or minutes, it all transcends to absolute, pure joy. When a momma sees and better yet holds her baby for the first time, the world changes. Her world changes.

Fast-forward a few, maybe many, years and possibly add a few more kids to the mix, and your struggle is redefined as searching for new ways to sneak veggies in the mac 'n' cheese and hunting down the nearest caffeine-rich beverage before the chaos unfolds. This was where I was when I wrote this. Not that my problems peak at things as trivial as these because that wouldn't be real nor relevant to inspiring anyone, including myself. But it's small things like trying to tote all forty-six grocery bags in your two arms, while holding a baby on your hip, unlocking the door, and not dropping the eggs, while in the rain; that can be the tipping point to total breakdown.

God has sent me my children to deliver me from my evil ways, I'm convinced. There's nothing that's revealed to me more about my lack than motherhood. I'd never described myself as angry until motherhood. I'd never describe myself as selfish until motherhood. I'd never describe myself as impatient until motherhood. Whether it's motherhood for you, a super-challenging job, an obligatory position you've had to take on against your will, or anything else that seems daunting, as well as totally beyond what you expected for your life, we all have opportunities to grow in humility.

Navigating motherhood has forced me to deal with my own memories of being a child and my relationship with my mother. As an adult child of divorce, I really didn't think I had issues regarding my parents' marriage or our family dynamics. At least I was an adult when my parents divorced. Those poor children who had to grow up with such brokenness…at least I was spared that. But as I've become more honest with myself, and with God, I've realized that there was always brokenness, major brokenness. My choosing to deny that simple fact or even minimize it holds me hostage to the dysfunction still relevant in my persona. And if there's anything I value, it's the need to be as functional as possible, Lord willing!

Humble beginnings

My life story is a lesson in humility. Characteristics of my life which point me back to humility have even just recently been revealed to me. I was a firstborn to spiritually lost and immature parents. Young and wild, my parents decided to change their ways when this pregnancy lasted longer than the first few. They married and had three more babies after me, exchanging a past full of irresponsibility for the American dream.

Growing up, I never questioned the normalcy of my life. I even esteem my parents for trading in their youth for us kids' futures. My parents were very involved in all our school happenings. They took me to sports and fun activities; they bought me a car when I turned sixteen; they assured me I could do whatever I wanted to do and be whomever I wanted to be. They did *many* things right, like introducing me to Jesus and church and paying for a private school education for several years. For those things, and much more, I'm forever thankful.

But our house was anything but orderly. We thrived on chaos. The status of my parents' marriage was always freshly reported to us kids or anyone within earshot. As the oldest and the only girl, my mom confided in me like a best friend. I have vivid memories of being called into the room to mediate arguments or testify against my dad on my mom's behalf. I remember feeling the need to counsel him on how to make Mom feel better and how to preserve the peace.

I have memories of holding my mom's sobbing face and stroking her hair as she lost herself in emotion on many nights.

Memories of my dad staying gone until the wee hours of the night, when I'd hear his truck finally pull into the driveway, and then chasing him down the stairs to tell him, "Goodbye and I love you" before he was gone again, wondering if he would stay gone this time...

Memories of my parents screaming at each other and always threatening to divorce...

Memories of locking me and my brothers in a room and distracting them while our parents destroyed each other with their words...

Dysfunction was the name of the game at our house. At one time, we had fifteen pets: four dogs, six cats, two ferrets, two gerbils, and one raccoon. Yes, a raccoon whose name was Boshaw. We were late for everything. We drove recklessly everywhere we went. We never had bedtimes. And we were always together. I have very few memories of being apart from my parents or my three brothers.

We lived on about three acres, with plenty of room for riding four-wheelers, building bonfires, and swimming in the pool. Other kids thought our home was awesome and rightfully so! We basically had no rules. The lack of boundaries combined with so many *toys* wasn't all that harmful until we became teenagers. Somewhere along the way, probably much earlier than I even recall, I became responsible. I proudly took the position of *mama hen* to everyone in our home.

Did my parents need me to wake them up on time to take me to school? No problem. Did my brother need his homework done? No problem. Did the groceries need to be put up? No problem. Did my brothers need to be reassured that mom and dad were not going to divorce? No problem. And while most of the time, actions like these weren't all *that* dysfunctional, it was the identity I found in being responsible for others that was. Far be it from me at the time, but that responsibility was only going to become *more* detrimental to my functionality as I grew up.

Taking responsibility became my coping mechanism for the chaos I couldn't control. If things were disorganized, messy, or combative, I could handle it. Any pain or disappointment manifested in me was something I questioned. Any pain or disappointment apparent in others around me, like my parents and brothers, was also something I questioned.

I dealt with things out of my control or beyond my understanding by taking responsibility for things that didn't have anything to do with me. Was there a way I could counsel my mom into being happy again? Was there something I could say that would make my dad give me his attention, or more commonly, give my *mom* his attention? Was there some way I could help or protect my brothers, so they wouldn't feel the same pain I did?

These were questions constantly swimming in my mind.

I later learned that I had become overresponsible, taking on other people's emotions and problems as my own. This made me feel like I had a purpose, like I could fix things like I could fix people. And that type of identity continued to grow in me until it was challenged in dating and marriage.

It's really hard for me to honestly recount the dysfunction of my family because I want to honor my parents. To honor them, I'm being discreet about some of the examples. They were doing the best they knew how at the level of spiritual maturity at which they were. All their actions were intended to demonstrate their epic love for us, and for that, I'm forever grateful.

But I also want to be perfectly clear. Being a Christian, loving Jesus, and wanting to do the right things are not enough. It wasn't enough for my parents. And later on, it wasn't enough for me. Looking back, it seems that neither of my parents focused on God as their sole source. My mom was chasing my dad for the love he didn't give; my dad was craving respect she didn't give and also just running from my mom chasing him; they both found their way back to us to fill their cups. We kids became the distraction and the center of that storm.

When I was going into my senior year of high school, my mom told me she and my dad were going to get on antidepressants. She

13

said she couldn't handle the thought of me leaving. She explicitly expressed how much heartbreak and hurt she felt at the thought of me leaving. One day, she'd be encouraging me to try out for a collegiate cheer squad, and the next day, she'd be begging me to stay home. She told me she couldn't handle me being gone. As the oldest of the kids and a first-generation college attendee, I was already freaked out about leaving at all. I was completely codependent on my family. They needed me. My mom needed me. How could I abandon her when for the last seventeen years, she's confided in me how much she needed me and how she's felt abandoned by everyone she's loved?

I remember as a teenager asking my mom if I could go to the mall with a few girlfriends.

"Why would you want to go without me?" she replied. "Can I go with y'all?"

My mom was the coolest. Of course, all my friends loved her. She was beautiful and funny and loved engaging us on our level.

"Um, yeah, I'm sure the other girls would think that was okay," I'd say.

"Well, if you don't want me to go, Amber, then I'll just stay home by myself."

I never saw this type of talk as manipulative, or guilt-driven. But this kind of interaction decorated our relationship for as long as I can remember. And of course, as I matured, bravely went off to college, and eventually got engaged, I became less and less codependent. And my mom became more and more dominant over me.

You see, my mom put me in the position that my dad should have been in. And more so, I was in the position God should have been in. I was her *person*. I was her only girl, the baby who turned her life around. I was the pregnancy that changed her life. I was there for her when my dad wasn't. I was there for her instead of hanging out with other kids my age. I stayed home instead of going to sleepovers. I went to her exercise classes and hung out with other adults her age instead of going to summer camp. For years, I found purpose in being her savior, and not just hers but anyone who needed saving.

This savior mentality really screwed me up for a long time. And to be honest, I still struggle to be free of it. I believed that to avoid feelings of shame and guilt, doing whatever it took to keep people happy is what made people love me. That's what made me lovable to God because I was being unselfish. Yet throughout my adolescence and young adulthood, I carried this burden to do the right thing, even if it meant being rejected by others.

The combination of wanting to please people and desperately wanting to please God landed me in a very isolated state of being for most of my young life. Reflection has shown me that God had called me even way back then to be set apart to serve Him in Christlike ways. But especially back then, that setting apart was so, so painful.

As a kid, everything is magnified. One person's slightly offensive RBF might have made me create a story in my head that they hated me, that they were better than me, and that I'd never fit in. This doesn't just go away as an adult either. How many times have you assumed that someone is rude or snooty when really, they were just completely oblivious to their resting face?

Which lies have you believed?

Humility comes when you realize you've been believing lies. These lies have directed your entire purpose in life, or lack thereof. The encounters of my adolescence that had any hint of rejection only reiterated the story I had told myself: my purpose is to save others, to be responsible for them. They're counting on me, and if I fail at all, or do anything that doesn't consider someone else's feelings, then I'm doing something horribly wrong. And they won't love me. God won't love me.

These patterns continued into adulthood, even after marriage. The dysfunction was really revealed to me after my parent's epic four-year divorce battle. Divorce became a reality for my parents after all of us were older than eighteen, and we began to have separate lives. Each of my parents spiraled in different ways. They each had reasons related to each other, but it still revolved around the idea that neither of their needs was being met, and they each were wounding the other over and over again.

One night, my husband and I were just about to leave my parents' house. It was late, and we were walking to our car. My mom had gotten mad at my dad over something, and she'd stormed out of the house, gotten in the car, and sped off. I went in to check on my dad, to see what happened, and he said she'd grabbed a gun, threatened him, and took off. I pleaded with my dad to take her seriously. But the reality was that this wasn't the first time she threatened to kill herself. She'd been known to drop the "You'll be sorry" line at either my dad or us kids. My dad was numb to it all.

My husband and I decided to call the police. I wanted to do whatever it took to preserve the peace, protect my family, and find my mom. They found her. They ended up taking her to jail and then transferred her to a psychiatric hospital. She stayed there for one week. That week, she'd call me, crying out for me to not abandon her. She asked me why she was there. She blamed my dad. She claimed he wanted to hurt her like this. She was freaking out.

But we knew it was out of our control. Although she accused my dad of *putting her there*, the authorities were obligated to keep her in the hospital because of evidence found that presumed she was trying to hurt herself or others. This instance was one of the first times I remember having such internal conflict between my reactive emotions and the wisdom I'd gleaned thus far.

So much of me wanted to drive to the hospital and break her out. But the wise part of me knew that I tended to enable her (and anyone) who was in pain. She had a reputation for making a scene or causing chaos anytime she became upset. Her lack of self-control contributed to me feeling the need to always be in control. Both ways are wrong.

When she got out of the hospital, she filed for divorce. Little did I know, this was the beginning of an abusive, psychological battle that would consume parts of my soul for the next several years.

The years that followed were full of text messages, voice mails, rants, and outrageous episodes of rage. Without thoughtful boundaries I'm currently enforcing, my present season would be filled with the same occurrences. My mom had made up story after story of how my dad and others were trying to silence her, harm her, steal from her, kill her, or kill me, etc. Accusations and theories involving my family members popped up like bubbles at the top of a diet Coke. Unlike a diet soda, it's a hard drink to swallow.

One night, I got a phone call from her, hysterical, telling me someone was coming to kidnap me. She adamantly cried out, "They're coming to get you, Amber. You have to do something. They're after you!"

One day, she showed up over here in a wig. Later on, she whipped off the wig to show me all her hair had been shaved. Her waist-length, thick, blond hair was gone. All of it. It was shocking. But not near as shocking as hearing that robotic bugs had crawled into her skin and poisoned her. They were still in her.

"Who did this to me, Amber? I know you know. Tell me, for God's sake, please!"

Once again, I was held responsible. And this time, I wasn't choosing to be in that position. She would put me there. And she'd put anyone who fit her bill there.

One day, she admitted to having taken methamphetamines. I thought I saw the light! A couple of weeks later, after she insisted she *was never* that *addicted*, she blew up my phone in the same kind of self-sabotaging spiraling for which she'd become known. She blamed me for her return to darkness. I was responsible for her pain. How could I do this to her?

There were many, many instances of abuse and manipulation and pure hatred translated through texts, outbursts, and voice mails. I credit God for covering me with a protective salve that's graciously defended me against some of the hateful curses aimed straight at my soul. But it's this abuse and these heartbreaking accounts that have moved me to understand how humility surfaces through desperation in light of God's Word.

Oh, how I desperately need Him. Oh, how I was so insufficient at defending myself. It became clear that I was totally out of control, and there was nothing I could do to help her anymore. And I honestly couldn't help myself without clinging onto a posture of pure humility in the depths of my soul.

> For the sake of Christ, then, I am content with
> weaknesses, insults, hardships, persecutions,
> and calamities. For when I am weak, then I am
> strong. (2 Corinthians 12:10)

Honesty about my past and where I've come from emphasizes humility in who I am. It's only by God's grace I am who I am today. No family is without some dysfunction. But here's the thing: God being the focus resets family to functional.

Humility in marriage

My husband and I celebrated ten years of marriage in 2020. Every year on our anniversary, I reflect on how far God has taken us since we started. Ask any married or divorced person, and they'll probably concur that marriage is *way* harder than you think before you get married. And my husband and I'd agree. It's been *way* harder than we ever imagined.

Despite witnessing my parents' troubled relationship, I, like most teenage girls, dreamed of one day falling in love and marrying someone who would always make me happy. Most of my preteen and teenage years were spent being the *supercool chick* with many guy friends. I was a cheerleader and a softball player. Remember, I lived at the *cool* house with all the boy toys. Usually, friends would come over and ask me to invite other girls over. I had crushes and boys I liked more than friends, but the story always ended with me feeling left out, rejected, used, and just not good enough. Many of these trivial moments translated into the lies of rejection I so quickly believed.

In response, I tended to put more effort into areas I could control and excel at like schoolwork, advanced classes, extra credit, and cheerleading. As I got older, I managed to create quite a reputation for myself, often being known as someone who always did the right thing and *never* did anything wrong. This totally twisted me up in my thinking about who I was and who I could be. It further disrupted the identity God had for me and made me rely on myself more than ever. Although I felt this deep sense of rejection down in my soul, I functioned as a confident young woman who appeared happy no matter what.

Everything I thought I knew about myself came to a pause when I fell head over heels in love with Micah Dobecka. He and I had been friends since our freshman year of high school and began dating my junior year. He was the first boy to express a desire for me and not just what my family, house, or freedom could provide him. Every detail about our togetherness seemed to fit perfectly.

His parents and my dad had grown up together and had a long family history. He played football and basketball, and I cheered for him on the sidelines. He adored the outdoors and had a four-wheeler of his own. He got along with all my brothers and was respectful of my parents. Once we began dating, we were inseparable.

We endured long-distance relationship struggles for a couple of years until we couldn't anymore. Micah left his university and moved closer to mine. He attended college nearby, and at one point, we lived in apartments that stacked on top of each other. We were having fun. And yet we were so dysfunctional.

I expected him to treat me like a wife, and I was trying to treat him like a husband. Not only was it inappropriate because we were not married but also because we'd never been modeled what a healthy marriage was supposed to look like. I so desperately wanted the peace that I thought would come from a healthy marriage, but I hadn't a clue what a healthy relationship looked like. We got engaged in my last year of college and married the summer after graduation. We were twenty-one years old and in some way the same fourteen-year-old kids we were when we met.

But you know what's funny? Other adults and people didn't have a clue. I don't remember anyone objecting to us marrying nor warning us of the challenges ahead. Maybe it was because we surrounded ourselves with people who had either failed in relationships or found their hope in ours. What I do know is that I was certain marriage was going to fix the fact I still felt rejected down deep in my soul.

Our relationship was littered with points of conflict that offended me. I felt constantly offended by Micah. When I'd try to explain how I felt, whatever I said translated to, "You're not good enough," to Micah. We each had massive wounds that needed healing. I kept holding my broken heart out to Micah to heal, and his response or lack thereof only made my wounds worse. It was never his fault. The fault for my pain was mine for looking to him as my source. He became *my* person.

Just over a year into our marriage, that wound of mine took over my mind, and I didn't even know it. I had let so much resentment and disappointment regarding Micah and my marriage build up, I found myself in the most vulnerable of positions. And once again, I was unaware of my vulnerability because I had always identified myself as someone who could never do anything wrong. Others had even agreed with me!

But I did. And since then, I've done many other things wrong. Early on in our marriage, I cut my husband down with my words and actions. I made him question my faithfulness. I made him question his identity as a strong man of God. Instead of nurturing the potential in Micah, in my pain, I pointed him to his problems. In my hurt, I hurt him.

Throughout these first few years, Micah started spending more time away from home, mostly because of his career. At first, I would punish him for that. As I grew in God, I slowly changed my response to him. I started disciplining myself to spend that alone time purposefully. As I learned to take my grief to God instead of my husband, I saw the alone time as an opportunity to intentionally anchor myself to the Lord. No longer would I crash back and forth like an emotional wave hitting the shore. I decided then and still daily to choose to steady my emotions by humbling myself before God.

Year after year, I've learned to see myself as the human I am not the savior I wanted to be. I've sought healing and humility through deliverance, Christian counseling, and mentorship at church. At my darkest points, I found myself in a bed of grief, considering suicide over my failures. I've punished myself far more than Micah ever had. He had so easily forgiven me for the ways I'd hurt him. I hope that I've gotten better at forgiving him (and others) as he did me. In the past, he's even reminded me of the scripture on redemption found in 1 Corinthians 10:13 on the card.

> No temptation has seized you that isn't common for people. But God is faithful. He won't allow you to be tempted beyond your abilities. Instead, with the temptation, God will also supply a way out so that you will be able to endure it.

That lowness I finally felt in myself years ago, that desperation, drew me to humility as I'd never known it. I broke. I realized I had already been so broken but had fooled myself into believing I could be perfect. I would never ever say that I'm glad we go through calamity, but I also have to wonder if I'd ever understand forgiveness, grace, and humility the same way if we didn't.

It's extremely difficult to describe the unraveling of who I thought I was, who I was to the love of my life and, in turn, to God. It's hard because it's humiliating to confess sins like pride, unfaithfulness, and lust. It's hard because the enemy suggests that talking about my sins will cause more pain to both me and my husband. It's not just *my* story. It's my husband's. But the truth is that bringing anything out of the darkness into the light is life-giving, not taking.

It doesn't matter what your sin looks like. The Bible says sin is sin; God sees it all the same. This is so hard to wrap our human minds around because we rate our sin as if some is worse than others. But all our sins should humble us in front of the extravagant grace God gives us.

Practicing patterns

Until we are made aware of our differences, we assume everyone is like us. We assume our family's completely normal until we're made aware they're not. We assume the way we think is right until we're proven wrong. This is part of maturity. And this is why humility as a foundational value is of epic importance.

After my husband and I came to a place in our marriage where there were no longer secrets and no longer misfired expectations of holding each other responsible for our pain, we became aware of the opportunity to establish a new legacy for our family. We liken it to planting a new family tree, with new godly roots, free of the bondage of our past. We'd hear songs like "Chain Breaker" by Zach Williams or "Break Every Chain" by Jesus Culture and get fired up about doing things differently.

Reflection allowed us to see the patterns of our past. We saw wounds, sin, and stories we believed that molded our minds to think the way we had thought for years. It gave us self-awareness that explained how and why we were the way we were. We clearly identified patterns in our past (abuse, sin, dysfunction, mindsets, etc.) that we didn't want to carry into our future. As I look back at the ways I was neglected as a child, verbally abused, spiritually abused, and modeled division through a family history of divorce, adultery, rage, and depression…all that helped me explain how broken I was and why. But knowledge isn't enough.

See, this knowledge in my personal life, while bringing me to a new level of humility and brokenness, could have kept me there—stuck in brokenness. This knowledge illuminated the areas where I, along with my ancestors, had failed in the past and could potentially fail again. The enemy used this knowledge as an opportunity to trap me in fear. That's why knowledge without truth is dangerous.

The truth that must not be left out is that God must be my champion. He has to be my source. It's only through Jesus that I've been given an opportunity to walk forward despite fear, along with the Holy Spirit. If I try to *will* myself into healing and freedom by knowledge alone, I will fail. It's only through the power of the Holy Spirit that I'm able to walk in the favor God has for me, which not only leads me into all truth, but also into peace, joy, grace, and abundance.

The Holy Spirit also empowers me to take authority as His daughter over these evil things (suicide, adultery, divorce, depression, rejection, abuse, etc.) and bring them to bow under the reign of Jesus Christ. I've learned that using this kind of language in my prayer life, especially when my emotions and mind start to take me adrift again, is how we walk in freedom and healing. Becoming free from the eternal consequences of sin happens instantaneously when we're saved. But becoming free from the power of sin happens gradually as we continue to commit our lives to Jesus through consistency in our spiritual disciplines.

CHAPTER 3

GRIEF

Saving what was lost

BEFORE I DISCUSS some of the spiritual disciplines that have equipped me to know God more and live healthier and freer, I have to address something we Christians don't like to discuss. We love to talk about the overcoming life of being a believer. We love talking about prosperity and grace and God's promises. But I've found that none of this positive chatter is relevant until I grieve what's lost.

Even Jesus Himself told His disciples that he had come to save what was lost (Matthew 18:11). After the fall of Adam and Eve and the entrance of sin's presence into the world, we lost something. God lost something. He lost His creation's perfection. He lost the love of His children and the opportunity to reveal Himself to them like He had. In Genesis, God walked and talked with Adam and Eve in the garden. They were in a perfect relationship. Adam and Eve were in a perfect relationship as well. They co-labored harmoniously. They didn't oppose each other but rather glorified God by reflecting His perfect image through their union.

After sin entered the world, we lost so much. We lost intimacy with the Father, intimacy with each other, and perfection of self. Throughout scripture, God expresses grief over this loss. He pleads with the people to be in a relationship with Him. Over and over,

His children rejected Him. People back then had the same issues we have now. They idolized other things; they idolized themselves; they sought pleasure instead of pursuing God. They didn't value God's presence nor understand the weight of it.

> The Lord was sorry that He had made man
> on the earth, and He was grieved in His heart.
> (Genesis 6:6)

But God, in His infinite wisdom and love, made a way for us to be restored to intimacy in our relationship with Him. He orchestrated the complex yet profoundly simple story of Jesus as Savior of the world. The complexity of God is relevant because we can see that from the very beginning, God had a plan to save us. He had a plan to restore us. The simplicity is found in that we don't have to do anything to earn this amazing gift of grace. We're redeemed simply by choosing to be in a relationship with Him.

Understanding the gospel like this helps me understand the importance of grief. As I've mentioned before, my pursuit of knowing God and going deeper with Him has revealed so much truth. I've recognized the truth of my own experience—what the real problems were, what the real dysfunction was, and what I've sacrificed and missed along the way.

To get physically healthy, I had to stop consuming junk and start feeding my body fuel. To get spiritually healthy, I've had to stop consuming lies and start feeding my mind truth. I've had to humbly own all my issues. But to move forward in the healing, I've also had to grieve some of the imperfections.

You see, discovering what's disappointed me for so long is not something you can just confess and move past. I've had to allow myself to experience the emotion of it. When I'm allowed to feel the pain, it becomes real. I can invite God to take it from me. If I never make it real, then I'm not fully surrendering it to my heavenly Father, who desperately wants me to cast my cares on Him. And if I expect to confess it once and not deal with it again, then I will fall into disappointment and self-loathing once again. My expectations for myself have to be decreased, and my expectations for God have to be increased.

Grieving the idea of self-perfection

> Therefore, I urge you, brothers and sisters, in view of God's mercy, to offer your bodies as a living sacrifice, holy and pleasing to God—this is your true and proper worship. (Romans 12:1 NIV)

For so long, I had just enough Jesus in my life that I believed if I worked hard enough and trusted God a little, then I could arrive at perfection. The only arrival at perfection is through a purely humble heart and reliance on the Savior. It requires no *hard work* as I had defined it my whole life. Nothing earnable or doable is involved in the equation. Anything I add to the equation is negative. But Christ covers whatever I take away to balance it out. I have to release any good thing I think I can offer to Him. This is what it means to be a living sacrifice. It's in the release that I surrender control. I must continually choose to see anything good I do or am as both a gift and an offering to Him.

This is a process. When I'm faced with the error of my ways, I realize that my dream of arriving at perfection is over. Confession leads to repentance and repentance leads to redemption. But this idea of perfection I had for so long requires no redemption, which once again omits any need for God. That's why it's so wrong to even subconsciously consider perfection as a destination in ourselves. We only arrive there through Jesus and upon entrance into Heaven.

What do I grieve?

In my experience, I've had to grieve ideas about marriage and family. I've had to grieve mistakes and the reality of regret. I have to grieve the energy wasted doing self-focused things and time spent thinking about worldly ways. I grieve attitudes and beliefs I've held that got me thus far, the ones I gleaned to, to protect myself and build myself up. I still grieve over the pain it caused me and the pain it caused the ones I love most. The very people I desperately wanted to please and protect were the ones that my striving for perfection hurt.

I've had to grieve the loss of control. Realizing that so much of my life's pain was caused by trying to cope and control is heartbreaking. Allowing myself to feel the negative, painful emotions instead of fixing them is hard. But I've learned I have to do it. I've cried about how weak it makes me feel to admit I can't do something to fix something or someone, but once again, that draws me back into a state of honesty and humility—right where God wants me to be.

Increasing intimacy with my husband has revealed how much distance developed from me trying to pull him closer to me. As a wounded wife, which we all are until we find healing and hope in Jesus, I handed my heart to my husband before I gave it to God. I grieve the time I wasted believing that it was his fault only. I grieve the time I wasted holding onto pain rather than apologizing for what I could and trusting God to handle the rest. I grieve the pain I've caused my husband by bringing so much pain and exposure to sin into our marriage. I have to surrender the regret of not healing and finding freedom before entering into the sanctity of marriage. And I choose to believe that God has healed me through marriage. I grieve the ways I pressured my husband instead of encouraging him, the ways I judged him instead of respecting him, and the ways I kept a record of wrongs instead of forgiving him.

I've had to grieve the speed at which I outgrew my childhood innocence. Parentification is what a counselor has called it for me. Becoming responsible for things that I should have never had to worry about caused me to not enjoy some parts of my childhood, remembering specific memories and feeling those faraway sensations of confusion, empathy, and loneliness again. Those feelings of rejection, responsibility, and regret are all streets I've had to revisit again and again but this time, with the Holy Spirit leading me and healing me along the way.

I've had to grieve the awakening of my sexual life through lust instead of love. Even though I lost my virginity to my future husband, we were not walking in His covering. Before even participating in sex, this lust had oppressed me since early, early exposure to sensual images and scenes from adult movies. I have memories of seeing things as early as five or six years old. I believe this added another layer of self-rejection. Any time I had thoughts about sex or before I knew what it was, just the images in my mind themselves, I felt dirty and ashamed. This opened doors to the spirits of shame and rejection to find attachment to me. I've had to grieve over the fact that this was neither my fault nor was it God's plan for me. I've had to grieve the time I've had to invest in gaining full freedom from this bondage.

I've also had to grieve the absence of adult parents. The brokenness caused by my parents' own struggles has affected my adult life and my kids. I don't have parents who babysit or wisely counsel us in our marriage and family. I don't have a mother who can safely be around my kids at all. My children won't get the sort of grandparent experience I always dreamed of having. They won't grow up visiting my childhood home and running through the same trails I ran through as a child. I've had to grieve the death of what I expected from my parents and yet still be hopeful for them to grow into their potential.

Receiving grace is key.

> But to each one of us grace has been given as
> Christ apportioned it. (Ephesians 4:7)

In the past year, I've realized how much I've still been trying to pay atonement for my sins. I've operated in a *works-without-grace* mentality. This is something else from which I've had to repent. I cannot pay back God for the sin or the harm I've done to others. I can't win back favor or trust. I can't pay my dues or receive enough punishment to wipe my ledger clear. Only the blood of Jesus can do that. What does that look like for me?

I must stop trying to please people and start understanding what it means to please God.

I must not try to elevate my own self-worth or self-image but instead trust God's truthful explanation of who I am as His child and His masterpiece.

I must not serve with selfish ambition but serve as an overflow of my love for God.

I must confess and repent from sin daily or as often as I can. When I search my own heart for something to purge, I'm reminded of my weakness and give God an opportunity to be strong on my behalf.

If I don't grieve over my loss, then I define myself as a savior.

There can only be one savior, and His name is Jesus (not Amber). I cannot save myself. No list of good deeds and no amount of humility alone can move me to redemption. When I tried to earn my way back or pay my dues, I was essentially convincing myself that I could somehow be the savior. I started to believe the lie that says, "I can fix it, I can fix myself, and I can fix the situation, and I can fix the other person." I judged myself and say, "If I can do *this*, then *this* will happen." And it either resulted in one of two postures:

1. I failed over and over so much that I began to think lowly of myself and hated myself. I allowed guilt, shame, and condemnation to identify me as worthless. I marked myself as unredeemable. A false humility became my badge. And no matter how much love others poured into me, I blocked the flow. I turned away from God. I clung to a badge called the *victim* and got stuck in a sinking boat of self-pity. I was so absorbed in myself that I blocked the face and loving embrace of God.

2. I thought that at some point, all the good I'd done paid my debt, and I'd earned my way back into deserving love. The moment I lied to myself and said, "I deserve or don't deserve something," was the moment I stopped receiving grace. I

judged myself and in turn, I started judging others. I allowed myself to hold others to certain standards. I rewarded them for good things, and I punished them for bad. I made others go through what I've put myself through. This could be something regarding my husband, kids, or anyone. This was pride because I was operating as if I were God. And if I was the one handing out grace or reward or punishment or judgment, then I would block myself once again from receiving grace. I turned away from God.

Grief can be present in a healthy marriage.

It's healthy to expect hard things, especially in marriage and family. One of the ways I fell into such dysfunction was by believing that a painless marriage was possible. Anything worth having is going to cost you something. I should have known this. I knew it to be true in fitness and nutrition and even in making certain financial investments. But I defined a good marriage as something free of struggle. I think part of me knew it was inevitable, but I wasn't capable of fighting fair nor functioning God's way if I felt like my husband was not also doing the right things.

"Why should I have to always do the right thing when it seems like he just does whatever he wants?" This was a question I arrived at during every argument or opportunity to humble myself before him and God.

The bigger question that seemed to rule my thoughts sounded more like, "Why do I always have to do the right thing? Am I not allowed to fall every now and then?"

These questions arose as I battled the insecurity of disappointing others. I elevated myself to a position that projected the pressure I put on myself as if it was placed there by others. I believed to fall was to fail, and to fail was the end.

Early on in our relationship, Micah and I fell into sexual sin: sex before marriage. Many people might say, "Well, yeah, but that's not the same, since you married each other." Let me tell you that it still caused many issues in our ability to attain true intimacy. God designed us to experience a type of intimacy with our spouse after making a covenant with them, as a representation of the covenant love we have with the Father. Any time we seek intimacy outside that covenant, we are accepting counterfeit intimacy. And there will be consequences.

In our teens, Micah and I awakened our sexuality through lust rather than love. And if we're honest, we would both admit that we had awakened our sexuality through pornographic images or scenes from R-rated movies, long before participating in sex with each other. The exposure to sex at such an immature level—and even if awakened at a *mature age*— if it's in a context outside the sanctity of marriage, will always lead to trouble.

Even after vowing to not have sex anymore in college, we struggled with lust and felt powerless to walk in unity with each other. We weren't having sex anymore, but the damage had been done without a true transformation from the inside out. We saw it as *broken rules* rather than fully understanding the sanctity of sex and why we'd want to wait. For me, I believed to abstain from sex until marriage was the right thing to do; it's what I was taught, and it's what the church taught. I knew sex was good and that it was good for married people. But to me, even though I knew Micah and I were not yet married, I knew we would be eventually, and I treated him as my husband. I sought him to fulfill my intrinsic, God-given desire to feel joy and value and purpose. The eyes of my heart were always upon him. On the throne of my heart, I placed Micah instead of God.

Because of this dysfunction, I believed that marrying Micah and for us finally being able to share intimacy in the bedroom would miraculously allow us to arrive at this state of contentment. I believed that adding this element to our relationship would solve the problem I was experiencing. That's why when we were married, I was so caught off guard by my disappointment. My discontent only multiplied in marriage because I was seeking something from my husband that only God could give me. I was using an earthly method to evaluate a spiritual emptiness. Neither Micah nor I could ever fully satisfy each other, even if we were experiencing a daily climax.

Now thankfully, God in His inexhaustible grace has redeemed our marriage and sex life in ways that have far surpassed my ideas of marriage. But the point is that it involved grief.

I've had to grieve over sin we both fell into, and the sinful actions caused by sinful thinking and believing lies. I've had to grieve over the purity of marriage we could have entered into, if we had not awakened our sexuality through lust and before that by someone else who introduced it to us as children. The fights, the arguments, and the feelings of isolation and misunderstanding can all indicate that if we had only done better, we would be better.

But what I love about God and His truth is that His purpose will prevail no matter what. I know as it says in Romans 8:1 that God works everything for the good of those who love God and are called according to His purpose. I know that my story would not be as relatable to others who have fallen in similar ways and therefore would not be as encouraging to some if I had not gone through the grief.

We also can't judge our past selves with the wisdom we have in our present selves. Of course, we'd do things differently if we knew then what we know now. But we didn't. And that's okay. God expects us to fail, and to grieve, and He's there with us every step of the way.

Grief produces desperation for God's wisdom.

Have you ever had one of those fights that have left you wondering if you're the crazy one? I've worn the badge for those types of battles for many years. Without inviting the Holy Spirit into these types of conversations, whether it be with someone else, or just a conversation in your head, you risk the opportunity for the enemy to trap you in shame, fear, and failure.

In my experience, the devil approaches me in my grief to accuse me of my past sin. He also accused whomever I have offense with of *their* sin and validates my sinful thinking. Without the Holy Spirit and engaging in this fight with God's power in me, I would be easily persuaded to side with the devil. He gets me to sit in a pity party, which only perpetuates my grief and draws me further and further from freedom.

However, I'm learning the value of spiritual disciplines like stopping periodically to pray. Once I've preemptively invited the Holy Spirit into my thought life, I've opened up the opportunity to use God's power to quiet the suggestions of the enemy. And when I obey in this way, my grief leads me to humility, which leads me to revelation.

Sometimes, I realize the error of my own ways or thoughts or maybe miscommunicated expectations. Sometimes, I realize that I have a wound from my past that was poked by an offense. Sometimes, I simply realize the goodness of God in that He quiets the screams of my soul when I turn to Him. He makes Himself known to me as bigger than my problems and my pain. My perspective of God is renewed and restored to clarity when I focus on Him rather than what's grieving me.

One of the revelations I've come to discover after accepting that God made my husband and me vastly different is the way we relate to others. Micah naturally lives guarded and keeps his heart to himself, offering small pieces out judicially. I give away my heart to everyone, without using discernment or discretion. Operating this way has indirectly devalued what I give to Micah.

For many years, I looked to Micah as the king of my heart. He ruled over my attitude. If I felt that he was upset with me, then I dropped everything to amend a problem that may or may not have even existed. My joy was dependent on him.

The essence of sin is seeing the creation (God's people and created things) as the answer to our heart's searching instead of seeing the Creator as the end-all, be-all King of our heart. The solution for each of us is to give our hearts completely to God, first and foremost. When we hand over our broken hearts to the Healer, He refines us and redeems us. He will equip us to give others a more complete, restored heart.

Grief repeats itself and reveals itself in different seasons throughout life's journey.

Something we have to accept for grief to be a positive part of our life is that it's something we must experience over and over again. Life is experienced in seasons, and with every season comes new challenges, new sin, and new grace. My sin is usually not a onetime bad choice. It's a series of thoughts and emotions that I nurture. It's a pattern of thinking which leads to actions. It's usually rooted in poor meditations, unholy recitations of things contradictory to God's truth. Most of the time, I don't realize I've been hosting an unholy mindset until some sort of action is born. It may surface as anger or screaming at my kids. Yep, that's usually the way it goes for me these days.

But it could also surface as depression or anxiety or lying to someone or hiding your emotions from someone, or filling your schedule with busyness to avoid being alone. We have to come to an understanding with ourselves that we are not good enough by ourselves. We need Jesus. We need all of God—the Father, the Son, and the Holy Spirit—to fill our souls so that He becomes our focus. When we focus on Him and allow Him to prompt us, motivate us, drive us, and correct us…even when grief attacks our thoughts and emotions, we can stay the course and come out stronger, wiser, and freer.

Sometimes our breakdowns result in God's breakthrough!

Grief is not a destination but an avenue that helps us arrive at humility. I mentioned this idea earlier, but experiencing pain and *really* feeling it can lead us to feel hopeless in ourselves. If we have the knowledge of the gospel, then we can remind ourselves that our hope is in Jesus and that we can do all things through Christ. This level of grief is a passing point. Desperation is not a place to be planted, but it is a place to grow.

> For though we walk in the flesh, we are not waging war according to the flesh. For the weapons of our warfare are not of the flesh but have divine power to destroy strongholds. We destroy arguments and every lofty opinion raised against the knowledge of God, and take every thought captive to obey Christ, being ready to punish every disobedience, when your obedience is complete. (2 Corinthians 10:3–6 ESV)

The acknowledgment of the hopeless state of ourselves can be a positive detour we must take for us to realize how we may have been operating independently of God's grace. It's in this part of grief where we must take our thoughts captive to the obedience of Christ. What does God say about what I'm thinking and feeling?

Too many people are identifying themselves solely on how they feel. There's a reason why people in this generation are desperate for acceptance and reject any sort of conviction. We have an unbiblical definition of love and acceptance and a worldly context to which we apply it. We now accept sin and shame as parts of our identity and forego the opportunity to surrender to the Healer and Creator.

If we were to see grief as an inevitable part of life and assuredly a part of a life surrendered to God, then maybe we'd be less inclined to believe discomfort and correction are bad. Jesus told His disciples that they'd experience trouble but to take heart. When we know this truth, we can overrule our thoughts and feelings that contradict it during times of grief.

Grief leads to healing, which leads to rest.

When I receive revelation, I feel alive. I feel like the wisdom I've experienced was worth the grief. I also sense God's presence in me and around me even in unfortunate circumstances. This, I believe, is evidence of the peace that passes understanding (Philippians 4:6). This peace is what we're all after. It's joy independent of our bank accounts, relationship status, or social media standing. It's the knowledge of love that drives me deeper than my feelings. This peace is what I'm after, most days, and most moments, especially in this current season of mine.

At the time I was writing this, I was pregnant with my third baby and often alone with my two boys under five years old during the aftermath of the COVID quarantine. Most days, to say, I lived exhausted feels like an understatement. But the exhaustion was more than just physical. It was an emotional, mental, and spiritual demand that felt like I'd never be able to supply.

But that's the point. I can't. I won't. Not without God.

> But he said to me, "My grace is sufficient for you, for my power is made perfect in weakness." Therefore I will boast all the more gladly of my weaknesses, so that the power of Christ may rest upon me. (2 Corinthians 12:9)

The rest we're all after is peace in our souls. I believe that in certain seasons, we'll experience more trials than others: more tests of our faith and opportunities for us to self-examine to discover how much we're depending on ourselves or others instead of God. But even in the seasons of chaos, we can carry on with rest. It's not a destination, but it's a ramification of our faith in God. Our eyes are open to the gifts of grace and rest as we transition ourselves into the passenger seat over and over again. Somehow, I keep finding myself behind the wheel—hey, Carrie—but God will never turn me down when I ask Him to switch seats.

When I admit in my grief that I need God, oh how I desperately need God, I'm essentially handing over my broken pieces to the Creator. It's in His nature to restore me to His original intent. His purpose for me is to be healed and set free. He will not leave me or forsake me. And His love never fails. I fail, but He does not. I can't, but He can. I won't, but He will.

This revelation of God's strength amid our suffering is something I pray we all learn and experience. I know so many have horrific pain in their past or even in their present. Maybe it's abuse or sickness or failure. Maybe it's a death of a loved one or a loss of a pregnancy. In no way do I want to minimize whatever struggle you face. But what I hope to do is point you to the author of all hope. I pray that just by reading my story and these words of mine, the spiritual doors open to God and close to the enemy. That your personal testimony of God's goodness is unveiled and put on display for you to see.

> *Lord,*
>
> *I lift up my brothers and sisters in Christ who are reading this book and plead with You, our perfect Father, Healer, and Redeemer, to do what only You can do. May You cover the pages before and after this passage with Your grace and anointing so that all who read may find inspiration to seek You and know You. Would You restore these loved ones to Your heart and mend the pieces of their own heart in ways that claim the redemption You promise us? Thank You that You love us and call us to both purpose and glory, as You provided for Your precious Son, Jesus. We trust You and believe You in Your word. We love You!*
>
> *Amen.*

CHAPTER 4

OBEDIENCE

I DON'T KNOW if I've ever thought about obedience more than now. Every day I struggle to discipline my children and teach them to obey. A new challenge awaits me every morning when it comes to the concept of obedience. "Oooooooobeyyyyyyy!" I preach to my children, and yet I can't just demand that they obey. I've learned I must explain what this command to obey means.

Understanding the notion that obedience must be learned requires a better understanding of our natural state. Just look at a child. They don't need to be taught to say no and don't need to be shown how to rebel or sin. It comes naturally, too naturally in my opinion.

Every choice to obey is something we must both demonstrate and implement to our children. We demonstrate obedience by humbly obeying God. When I'm transparent to my children, apologize when I'm wrong, and explain how I'm trying to obey God's command of me as a grown-up and a mommy, I'm demonstrating obedience. When I proactively express an expectation for my kids' behavior and attitudes and discipline them for not doing what I know they're capable of doing, I'm implementing obedience.

The obedience concept with children is one in progress, of course. And one I'm learning through trial and error. Yet one of the most profound lessons I've learned in trying to teach obedience is how disobedient I can be to my heavenly Father. Fits of anger and disproportionate reactions accompany my own disobedience. A loud—very loud—voice and smoke coming out of my ears (okay, not really, but it can feel that way) are evidence of this disobedience. When I'm obedient, I can live in peace of mind, even if my circumstances are anything but peaceful.

"When you don't obey, you will not play."

This has become a mantra in the Dobecka house. But I bet we can apply it to more than just the rewards of a child's playtime. God required obedience from His people in the Old Testament because the first covenant required perfection and completion of the law. In our sinful nature, we humans were unable to keep our side of the covenant. In turn, our loving Father sent Jesus, His only son, to fulfill our part. This upheld His fully just character and still allowed His children to be redeemed in the fullness of His grace. Now we obey out of love for our Father, not out of obligation. Our obedience is love-based, much like I strive to teach my own kids.

> And this is love, that we walk according to his commandments; this is the commandment, just as you have heard from the beginning, so that you should walk in it. (2 John 1:6)

The Bible is God's love story, where every page highlights how much He loves us and points us to Jesus, by whom He demonstrated that epic love. When we read the Bible with this in mind, we can see past the commands and see it as a guidebook to truly being a reserve for peace and love and all the fruit of His spirit.

> But he said, "Blessed rather are those who hear the word of God and keep it!" (Luke 11:28)

Much in the way I want to teach my children godly character so that their hearts are pure, God wants His children to be more concerned with the heart also. The Bible has many examples of what it means to be obedient in your deeds but disobedient in your heart.

I'm sure there are countless people, even some readers, who have found this to be true with those they've experienced in the church. Hypocrisy is rampant in that it's just so, so easy to appear righteous without having the character to back it up. I believe this has caused many people to turn their attention from the Bible, the church, and anything to do with God.

> If you keep my commandments, you will abide
> in my love, just as I have kept my Father's com-
> mandments and abide in his love. (John 15:10)

To me, this only causes more of a sense of urgency to share my personal love story with God. It amplifies my desire to both transparently and truly testify to the truth of His hold on my life. And if I'm to be transparent with others and myself, I must be able to face the places of my life where I've been disobedient, if even only in the posture of my heart. There are times I should have worshiped, and instead, I scrolled. There are times God was calling me to be still and instead, I made myself busy. There are times I should have apologized, and instead, I kept a record of wrongs. It's not that we should trap ourselves in shame, but we should allow conviction to move us toward graceful redemption through obedience.

> Do you not know that if you present yourselves
> to anyone as obedient slaves, you are slaves of the
> one whom you obey, either of sin, which leads to
> death, or of obedience, which leads to righteous-
> ness? (Romans 6:16)

The Bible makes it clear that if we're not being obedient to God, even if only by ignoring Him, we are obeying the father of this world, the devil. Many try to justify their choices by simply honoring their heart or claiming they're following their gut. But if our guts are not submitted to the authority of Jesus, then they're being swayed in the wrong direction. In Jeremiah 17:9–10, God says our hearts are sick and can lead us in the wrong ways. Like a child, we are born into sin and by default, we make selfish decisions that do not usually exhibit God's love. I don't mean to make some theological claim that we are all inherently evil and bad but only to urge us all to fully examine our value of godly obedience.

Questions to ponder:

- *How do my actions support that loving God is my first priority?*
- *How do my thoughts support that loving God is my first priority?*
- *Which experiences can I recall that reflect God's faithfulness to my obedience?*
- *What was the last thing the Holy Spirit told me to do that I haven't done?*
- *Is there something the Holy Spirit is convicting me of regarding obedience or disobedience?*

How are your habits?

Habits reveal so much about us. I have a really bad habit of leaving one last drink in all my beverages. I'll pour a cup of iced tea and leave two swallows worth in the pitcher. Or I'll make a pot of coffee and only drink half of it but forget to put the rest in the fridge. It annoys my husband so much!

At one point, I had a habit of waking up and working out every day at 5:00 a.m. Then the seasons changed. I had another baby, left the professional fitness world, and kicked the habit.

At another point, I had a habit of eating a bowl of cereal at least once a day. Usually it was in the morning, but sometimes, it was late at night. During a healthier time of my life, the bowl was full of Bran Flakes and All-Bran, but before that, it was Cinnamon Toast Crunch.

At another point, I had a habit of watching *Saved by the Bell* every day after school and dreamed of meeting Zack Morris in front of my locker.

Isn't it strange how habits come and go during different seasons of our life? Usually, habits are formed before we've consciously made an effort to identify them. They're the things we do without thinking. They're also the things we expect to occur no matter what else happens. We all have both good and bad habits, but considering them can give you insight into your mindset, your beliefs, your values, and whether or not you're obeying God.

God warns us against habitual sin. I believe He does so because He knows that we all fall short of perfection, and we're all going to make mistakes. But He also gives us what we need to know to make choices with Him in mind. This is why having positive habits and spiritual disciplines like reading the Bible, prayer, worship, and church are simple but so important to walk in obedience to God.

What do you believe?

For the majority of my life, I strived to always do the right thing. Although it poked my wound of rejection, most of me wore a badge of honor when people teased me about being a *Goody Two-shoes*. I felt like if I could work to never hurt anyone and make sure people were impressed by my willingness to do the right things, then I was obeying God. I knew just enough about what the Bible said from several years of Christian schools and attending church to reassure myself that as long as I did the right thing, I was okay. My head knew Jesus, but my heart never knew Him down to its depths. And you couldn't see His grace or power in my habits.

My old habits actually revealed how I believed I was responsible for my righteousness, not Jesus. This belief elevated my values for making people happy and improving myself in ways that could make people more happy. I believed if I could keep people happy, then God would be happy. But all that work to please people left very little time to do the few things God asks us to do.

I found myself only reading the Bible, worshipping, or praying when I was in church, in fear, or in pain. Coping with a deep wound of rejection and overresponsibility built a huge stronghold for self-righteousness, self-dependence, and self-focus. If I couldn't make myself loved by someone, or I felt misunderstood by someone, I broke. If manipulating language and oversharing didn't work to get them to see me from the angle I wanted them to, then I would come back to that growing wound of rejection and self-loathing.

Something's wrong with me. I'm not doing enough. I'm not being enough. They don't see me. They don't hear me. They don't love me.

I had a habit of using God when I felt I had nothing left to do. At those low points, I glorified Him as the Healer, the Savior, I knew I needed. But as soon as situations turned around, I abandoned God. I essentially said, "Thanks, God. Okay, I'm good now."

> Create in me a clean heart, O God, and renew a right spirit within me. Cast me not away from your presence, and take not your Holy Spirit from me. Restore to me the joy of your salvation, and uphold me with a willing spirit. (Psalm 51:10–12)

There came a time when I could no longer push God away. I became so broken down and disappointed over and over again in my attempts to control the way I felt (or desired to feel). I think I took my pain seriously when I admitted to having suicidal thoughts. I discovered that to find peace again, I had to fully know God and fully receive Him into my heart. I could no longer wait to welcome Him when I convinced myself I couldn't handle it. I needed to admit that without Him, I could never handle it. I needed to study His nature with this new perspective regarding my brokenness.

Instead of looking at God from the mountaintop I and others had placed myself, I found God from the pit I had fallen into. And this was the first time I saw God as big and powerful as He always was. In humility, I had to confess to God the error of my ways much like a daughter admits to her parents of disobedience. And just like a good Father, He embraces all His children with open arms and wisdom to correct. When I was honest with myself and God, I learned God's character by experiencing His presence. To continue to know God, I had to start applying discipline to my spiritual life as well as I'd managed in other areas.

> Do not be conformed to this world, but be transformed by the renewal of your mind, that by testing you may discern what is the will of God, what is good and acceptable and perfect. (Romans 12:2)

The Bible says God's kindness leads us to repentance (Romans 2:4). Knowing God as kind and good causes us to want to be honest with Him. It causes us to yearn for transformation. He gives us the ways to transform in His commands, the stories He includes in the Bible, and the whispers He speaks to us throughout the day. The more we know God as kind, good, and graceful, the more humble we become. This humility leads us to obedience, and obedience ignites the process of healing. As we're healed and set free, we can disciple ourselves and others into experiencing the power and joy and love of the Father.

Practicing discipline in small steps

> Motivation gets you going. Discipline keeps you growing. (John Maxwell)

Have you ever been on a diet? Or maybe made a New Year's Resolution? Or have you ever fasted and found out you're not as spiritual as you thought you were? Have you found that the fire you begin with goes out as time goes on? I'm raising my hand to all these.

Working on my own fitness and health, as well as coaching countless individuals, I've come to the conclusion that motivation is fleeting. The simple fact is that there are some days you're just downright unmotivated. Motivation is tied to your emotion. When you first commit to something, you tend to be more motivated because it's new and the hope of the unknown is exciting. Then you get started and realize this thing is hard, and your emotions change. What happens then?

Sometimes you have to do what you don't want to do. Discipline is doing the things we don't feel like doing because we know they're the right things to do. President Abraham Lincoln said it's choosing between what you want now and what you want most. Discipline is the activation of your free will and the alignment of your actions and thoughts to what you want most in life. It requires habit. It requires a pattern of thinking and doing—thought to action, mind to muscle. That's why physical disciplines like exercise, fasting, sports, dieting, etc. are all applicable areas of cultivating discipline.

Discipline begins in the mind. Once you have your *why*, or your initial motivation defined, you can easily filter all thoughts and feelings to either align with it or dismiss it. Truly, discipline goes hand in hand with mindfulness. For a while, the term *mindfulness* was all abuzz on Instagram, especially among fitness bloggers. Trainers would encourage others to become more mindful of their body, their worth, and their desires. It became one of those concepts that sounded good to mention but, on the surface, left you very shallow with nothing to do about it. For me, being mindful of something is equivalent to being intentional about it—thinking about it and pausing on that thought before moving to the next.

When I was about twenty-eight weeks pregnant with my second son, I ran into some issues with my lower back and hips. This led to an acute, debilitating pain in my right knee. I remember I was in the middle of teaching one of my cycle classes, and suddenly my knee felt like it had been stabbed with a railroad spike. It turns out my isolated knee injury was not that isolated. It had begun with overuse of my muscles in my glutes and quadriceps (my butt and thighs). Turns out, growing a baby, teaching ten-plus classes a week, and driving ten-plus hours a week create the perfect storm for an injury.

The thing was that taking a few days off exercise is a really big deal for me. It wasn't just my job, but it was my time of mental restoration. It was my *me* time and my time with God. As I scrambled to catch up on all my physical therapy and recovery exercises, I realized how *mindless* I had become when it came to exercising my body. I had gotten into a habit of going through the motions of exercises and increasing intensity without proper recovery, stretching, and reflection. Although the problem was created over time and through a process, the evidence of the problem arrived in an instant.

If I had proactively tuned in with my changing body, and given it the recovery I knew it needed, even though I didn't feel like it needed it at the time, then the bigger problem could have been avoided. I could have prevented weeks' worth of pain and hours' worth of foam rolling, stretching, and icing my muscles—not to mention the mental agony.

Episodes like this remind me to be more self-aware. Joyce Meyer says it like this, "Have you thought about what you're thinking about?" Becoming self-aware leads to a deeper understanding of your habits and the triggers that currently rule your actions or lack thereof. It also positions us to gain healing and freedom from the things that are keeping us in spiritual bondage so that the disciplines we form are actually fruitful. For me, at that time, I had a bad habit of trying to do too much and waiting until something in my body hurt before I stopped or recovered. I was doing all the right things but doing them from a position of unhealthy posture, so I wasn't really progressing; I was actually causing more stress.

> Search me, God, and know my heart; test me and know my anxious thoughts. See if there is any offensive way in me, and lead me in the way everlasting. (Psalm 139:23–24)

In the same way, we can be physically mindful, we can become holistically self-aware. When you spend time reflecting on what's going on in your mind, you become more self-aware. When you're self-aware, you can confess your need for the all-powerful God of the universe to come into your little universe. The discipline of confession brings us back to the importance of humility. We can't get there without it. Through a humble heart, we can examine our habits, routines, thoughts, feelings, memories, and triggers. The more self-aware you are, the more likely you are to know what to correct or change in your thinking, thus enhancing your overall discipline.

How do you start having a disciplined mind?

You start small. Begin with your daily agenda. And begin the night before. If you're like me, stress attacks the moment you awake, so discipline takes strategy. At night, I talk to myself about how my morning is going to go. I tell myself that the moment my eyes open, I'm going to think, *Lord, thank You. Help me today.* That way, my mind is immediately pointed toward a bigger purpose and a bigger source. It's a good idea to prioritize time with God first thing in the morning, even if that means you merely think, *Holy Spirit, help me,* before you get out of bed.

If you don't steer your mind in the direction you want to go, it will sway in whatever direction the winds blow.

I operate best when I feel productive. It's in my personality. But I believe we all feel better when we feel like we've accomplished *something*, even on our worst days. That's why I've found it helpful to turn trivial tasks into disciplines. Examples include making my bed when I wake up and cleaning up the kitchen before I go to bed. Now I totally understand that sometimes, these tasks can be considered things that either steal our joy or excuses for not tackling the bigger tasks. There should be times when these things are not the end-all and be-all of your identity. Sometimes, I also have to remind myself that just because it's noon, and I still haven't brushed my teeth, I'm not a failure.

That being said, I've personally found that even on the days I feel like I was busy all day and got nothing done, I found joy in wrapping up these small details. They probably look different for everyone. The point is to identify a few small things you missionize every day.

> Show yourself in all respects to be a model of
> good works, and in your teaching show integrity,
> dignity. (Titus 2:7)

This is a great place to start being more mindful. As you go about your day, take inventory of marks you're missing, but do so from an improvement mindset. As I find places I want to improve, I try to keep a record. I like to make a list of daily tasks and set it up where I can clearly see it all day, whether it's a list on my phone, a notepad, or a dry-erase board. I also hold myself accountable for a couple of trivial tasks like refilling the empty toilet paper rolls and cleaning off the tables. While these tasks may be things you think you already do with excellence, I'm sure you can find some other household tasks that require discipline. Examples include the following:

- meal prepping ahead of time
- writing down grocery-list items before shopping
- putting dishes in the dishwasher
- folding laundry and putting it in the drawers/closets
- replacing the toilet paper on the roll
- wiping away crumbs from the table
- waking up and going to bed on time.

> Whatever you do, work heartily, as for the Lord and not for men, knowing that from the Lord you will receive the inheritance as your reward. You are serving the Lord Christ. (Colossians 3:23–24)

You can also be more mindful of doing one small task at a time instead of feeling overwhelmed by a whole project. The point is to prepare what you can to avoid impulsive decisions. Anyone and everyone have something to steward, so either start with what matters to you most or what you can confidently accomplish.

In whatever season you're in, whether you're a young professional, student, parent, grandparent, or widow(er), some things must be done and people who need to be touched. If you still have breath in your lungs, God has a purpose for you. To truly understand His specific purposes, we must do our best in the day-to-day tasks especially because this is how we learn how to implement self-awareness and self-control, leading us to become a more humble vessel of God's power and love.

Spiritual disciplines don't have to feel spiritual.

In all my experience training others and myself, I've always found that agreement on a game plan is essential to success. It sets me and the client up with an understanding of the strategies that must be practiced to achieve the desired results. When the client is honest with me about their habits, beliefs, and desires, I can create a game plan that fits who they are and who they want to be. When the client trusts my expertise as the trainer and does what I've suggested, they will be successful. This is a simple illustration, but it correlates to the way God trains us.

He gives us a rule book with commands about righteousness, salvation, eternity, and peace on earth. The Bible is filled with true accounts about people just like us who either chose to trust God or not. They either walked in obedience or not. This book is also a beautiful word story of who God is and what he desires for His children. Every spiritual discipline I've tried to live out in my own life and would encourage others to do is rooted in the Bible and what it tells us to do. And many of these disciplines rely on a belief that the Bible is 100 percent true and inerrant.

1.   *You must agree with the Author of truth about who you are and who He is.*

One of the most popular topics for discussion in today's world is identity. Every person has a point in life where they feel like they need to suddenly become the person they're going to be for the rest of their life. The pressure to become that person is like a balloon on the brink of popping. How much air can you blow into it? How many titles, hobbies, talents, gifts, certifications, schools, and achievements can you fit onto your IG profile? How can I label myself to appear good enough?

And from a different aspect, what does my experience in life tell me about who I am? If I have experienced abuse, division, or neglect in my childhood experience, I might see myself as a victim and see others as untrustworthy or toxic. Or I might become codependent and seek to please others to find love and acceptance. If I've been hurt in a relationship or abandoned, I might become overly independent of others and avoid asking for help. There are limitless conclusions we arrive at regarding how we identify ourselves and others, and most of them are drawn from what we believed to be true based on our experience. This is how I'd describe what people in our culture now refer to as "your truth."

Today's culture celebrates everyone's *truth*. We force each other to accept whatever experience has taught us as individuals to be loving and affirming. The world says everyone has their own truth, and if your truth contradicts someone else's, then it causes division. This *acceptance of everyone's truth* is actually a rejection of the *real* truth.

My truth lies to me every single day. *My truth* tells me I'm responsible for sustaining other people's peace. That if I can make sure others are undisturbed, then I will be at peace. My truth tells me that when I feel like people don't love me, that it's possible to earn their love by doing more of what they want, even if it costs me. My truth tells me that to make a mistake is life-ruining, that to make someone uncomfortable is to hurt them, to break them, and that it's the most selfish, unforgivable move I can make. It tells me to be perfect is to be right and to be right is to be perfect. It beckons my heart to stay trapped in the stories I've told myself. The stories suggested I could control things or understand things, to understand why I felt broken and why others feel pain. It fools me into staying put, staying stuck, not progressing in freedom, but instead, accepting where I'm at. My truth affirms all the hurt I feel and tells me it's okay. My truth can even blame others and rule them guilty. But at its worst, my truth can blame *me* and rule myself guilty for a lifetime. And that's why my truth has to go.

I will replace my truth with the only truth that shall sustain me. That through Jesus Christ alone, I am saved. I cannot save myself nor save others. That this saving is not one and done but that the freedom of knowing the truth is more than just knowledge. It's knowing the Creator of knowledge. It's a process of reflection, revelation, and discipline. My truth has taken me captive for too long. I'll burn the truth that was actually a pack of lies all along! And I'll joyfully step into the identity God created for me, wild and spirited and deep and free.

So the first discipline is a commitment to the truth, not *your* truth but *His* truth. It might mean you need to simply read through the Bible, talk to a counselor, or join a group, but discover who God is and what He really says.

2. *You must love with your whole heart, mind, soul, and strength.*

Corporate worship has always been something that I've easily enjoyed. I loved the music and singing and the act of performing—well, obviously, performing because it aligned with my wounded heart about working for God's attention. But even despite having intentions that were slightly off, worship has always moved me.

Worship became real though, when I began worshiping on my own, in my personal time. Devastation about life brought me to a place of desperation. I think the season of life that taught me the power of worship the most was the season of infertility. After five years of marriage and never taking a birth control pill, my husband and I found ourselves ready for kids (at least we thought we were ready—hah). There was no way to try harder than we'd been trying, especially because I had amenorrhea (lack of menstrual cycles).

Years of overtraining and undereating took their toll on my body. No woman wants to complain about not having a period until you need it! At the time, I was teaching a Sunday cycle class, where the playlist incorporated worship music. Five minutes before class, I'd pray, "Holy Spirit, You're welcome here. Speak through me and minister to every person in this class." In each class, I surrendered to God with every exhaustive breath and pointed all to Him as the central focus. I had no idea how this simple routine would change my life forever.

The Holy Spirit began to move in each class. I felt empowered as I led on stage. Words would drip out of my mouth as fast as the sweat dripped off my skin. There were multiple testimonies of people hearing things I'd said over the microphone that resonated with them; they'd say it was just what they needed to hear. The kicker was that I didn't even remember saying these things! I began to journal my prayers and heart songs after class. I started implementing this approach in every class I taught—praying for the Holy Spirit to move beyond my physical movements.

Breakthrough met me in the deepest parts of my heart. I felt God whispering to me how much He loved me. Words can't express what I felt and knew in my heart, but I knew that no matter if I never had children, God loved me, and I loved Him. A couple of months later, I found out I was pregnant.

Imagine the excitement as I shared this news from the podium with all those who powerfully worshiped alongside me. Once again, God's power through the process was put on display. The simple discipline of praise inspires others to persevere through their own pain.

3. *You must pray as if you're talking to your best friend all day every day.*

Many of us grow up in church and understand the normalcy of praying in church, before meals, and before bed. But many of us didn't grow up witnessing parents who prayed unceasingly. Many of us had more negative influences on us than positive ones. And that jeopardizes our belief that prayer is normal and that prayer works.

When I was growing up, my mom would pray vivacious prayers. Oftentimes, she'd start praying in tongues. My dad hardly ever prayed. I remember my mom picking fun at my dad when he'd try, and say things like, "Oh, I guess he would know how to pray better if he prayed more often." I saw two extremes at work, and neither one looked right.

> Trust in the Lord with all your heart, lean not on your own understanding. In all your ways acknowledge Him and He will direct your paths. (Proverbs 3:5–6)

What I've learned as an adult is that the people who I want most to be like are the ones who normalize prayer and make it a part of their daily experience. I can begin a conversation with God from the moment my eyes open in the morning. "Holy Spirit, You are welcome here. Please help me today."

The conversation continues as I drag my feet to the coffee pot and carry crying babies. "Lord, I need You. Help me. The joy of the Lord is my strength." If the Holy Spirit is my best friend, He hears my thoughts and desperately wants me to ask Him to help me. He's a gentleman and will not take something from me unless I give Him permission. He wants to be acknowledged. He is soft-spoken yet powerful. And the more I bring Him into my daily thought life, the more power I give Him, which in turn empowers me.

> Do not be anxious about anything, but in every-thing make your requests to God…by prayer, thanksgiving and placing your request to God, the peace of God will guard your heart and mind fully beyond understanding. (Philippians 4:6–7)

I've learned to catch myself mid-complaint and turn it into a prayer request.

Lord, I'm so exhausted. I never get a full night's sleep anymore. Please help my children sleep peacefully and reveal any strategy I can implement to help us all sleep.

God, it feels like my husband doesn't listen to me when I ask him to do this or that… Please help me to not be so offended and please speak to my husband about this so that we are unified and so that I can love him and respect him. Please help me to speak to him with respect and not nag at him.

Father, I feel like my life doesn't matter, that no one sees me or cares about what I do. Nobody ever thanks me, and I have to do everything with no help… Please help to change my feelings and notice when others value me and love me. Please reveal your purposes for me in this season and protect me from the mental and emotional attacks of the enemy on my self-worth.

These are all examples of how to turn a normal feeling or thought into a prayer request that invites the power of the Holy Spirit. You can *think* of your prayers. You can speak your prayers out loud. You can pray with others. You can write your prayers. You should do all these things. But don't ever stop praying.

4. *You must meditate on God's Word as if you will die without it.*

For some reason, reading the Bible is the hardest of the spiritual disciplines for me. It probably means that in this season, it's the one in which God wants me to grow. Attending a Christian elementary school and a Christian university, I always felt like I knew the Bible. Knowledge of the Bible is dangerous because it invites a spirit of pride and complacency. Something that shakes me up is knowing that even Satan and his demons know the Bible. They have more scripture memorized than many Christians! The key is not just memorizing the verses, rehearsing the stories, or being familiar with the concordance, but it's knowing how to use the Bible as a weapon.

> For the word of God is living and active, sharper than any two-edged sword, piercing to the division of soul and of spirit, of joints and of marrow, and discerning the thoughts and intentions of the heart. (Hebrews 4:12)

To me, the Bible has an edge that God uses to pierce our flesh. God's Word sharpens us and sculpts us to become more Christ-like and holy. Sanctification is the process of right living that includes meditating on scripture. We are to know the Bible to convince ourselves of the truth and to discern God's will.

This sharp weapon can also defeat evil. Jesus used God's Word to defeat the temptation of Satan in the desert, when He remarked three different times, "It is written…" In John 17:17, God's Word is referred to as the truth. We can use God's truth to discover the thoughts we have that may be falsely accusing us, others, or even God.

> All Scripture is breathed out by God and profit-
> able for teaching, for reproof, for correction, and
> for training in righteousness. (2 Timothy 3:16)

His Word is not only meant to be our rule book, guidebook, and lifestyle map, but it's also meant to be a mode of personal communication with us. When we invite the Holy Spirit into our walk through the Bible, our minds are opened to the meaning of things that we otherwise might not understand. We might catch a theme or a word in a scripture that answers a prayer or leads us to make a decision we were anxious about. In Psalm 12:6, it says that God's Words are as flawless as purified silver and refined gold, so we can always count on His Word to be true and valuable.

> For everything that was written in the past was
> written to teach us, so that through the endur-
> ance taught in the Scriptures and the encourage-
> ment they provide we might have hope. (Romans
> 15:4)

Since the Holy Spirit wrote the Bible (inspired the human writers), we can trust that the scriptures are all supporting His main message: that He loves us. Reading the Bible gives you hope; it's encouraging. If you've ever read the Bible, and it's only challenged you, I'd recommend praying and inviting the Holy Spirit to guide you into all truth. What is He saying to you personally? If it's challenging you, maybe God is trying to change you, and it's okay if change is hard. It's meant to be hard.

For me, the challenge is in prioritizing the time and not procrastinating it. I find myself wanting to read other books or basically do anything else other than sitting down and reading my Bible. But I'm aware of the fact that those hesitations are not from God but from the enemy who is trying to do whatever it takes to keep me from rising toward my potential in God. The devil knows that if I read my Bible, I will know the truth, and I will be awakened to the power available to me.

He also knows that I have a whole list of excuses and really good reasons why reading my Bible is not as urgent as other things. And that brings it back to discipline. None of these things are easy. None of these things are natural in our flesh. But when we use discipline to consistently see ourselves and therefore, operate, as the spiritual beings we were created to be, we can do it.

5. *You must get involved in a church and be a part of the community there.*

We are social creatures, no doubt about it. As the world changes, our social interactions change, but it doesn't negate them all together. We thrive in relationships, and progress is made faster when we cooperate. There's a reason why the church, marriages, and family dynamics are under attack in our governments, politics, and social stigmas. It's because the devil is a liar, and he's been lying to people about what works and what doesn't work for centuries.

> The thief comes only to steal and kill and destroy.
> I came that they may have life and have it abundantly. (John 10:10)

Much like a lone sheep is prey for the wolf, a lone Christian is a prey for the devil. Depression, suicide, anxiety, and social disorders are prevalent in environments where people are abandoned or isolated, or at least when they feel that way. When you believe that you're more powerful when you're a part of a group, you release the burden of attitudes like pride, being judgmental, cynicism, narcissism, and self-pity. It's humble to accredit value to others, and humility is where all power begins.

I believe God refers to His children as sheep because He wants us to see that without a shepherd and without being a herd, we are the perfect prey for the enemy. We, as humans, and as God's children, require community for protection. We need to lean on each other sometimes. We're not meant to do life alone.

No other season of my life has taught me these values like being a firefighter's wife and mom to littles during a pandemic. Being a stay-at-home mom can already feel like you're trapped in your own home, often being a slave to a child's sleep schedule and feeding times, not to mention the child's attachment to everything *mommy* so that when well-meaning others try to help, it only causes more stress. I know the pandemic and the in-home orders affected everyone in some way, but for me, it really made me realize how necessary being around others is. Being present with others is not the same as having screen time with them. It's just not.

God created us with five senses, and He meant for us to use them all in relationship. When we can't hug each other, hold hands, and share food, we are not fully functioning in the community we're meant to be in. We each have a unique value we add to different circles and our gifts come alive in different communities.

> And let us consider how to stir up one another
> to love and good works, not neglecting to meet
> together, as is the habit of some, but encouraging
> one another, and all the more as you see the Day
> drawing near. (Hebrews 10:24–25)

A concern I have post-pandemic is that those believers who did not understand the power of congregating together in the church corporately will remain in their homes watching a church service on a screen. I'm concerned that many Christians who are destined for abundant living will find themselves doing religious things and checking boxes like *watch church* and not *be* the church.

Like Proverbs 27:17 says, "Iron sharpens iron," we all are meant to challenge and encourage each other. When you surround yourself with people who can help you and people who need to be helped, you will find purpose and power in the church.

You can't do it all with 100 percent effort.

As a recovering perfectionist, I want to emphasize this truth when it comes to implementing spiritual disciplines. It's totally acceptable to focus on growth in one area for a while and then growth in another area later. Even though I'd debate that some of us can multitask all day, I also have to admit that none of us can do everything with 100 percent effort.

There are times in my life when I focused on energizing my prayer life. I've made prayer lists and spent most of my quiet time thinking, writing, and speaking my prayers to God. Then there are other times I've spent my energy worshiping and thanking God, in song, and in meditation. It really comes down to what your intention is for that time.

With any intention to seek the heart of God, He honors it and loves it. So whichever discipline you spend time improving, remember that this walk with God is just that—a walk, not a run, and definitely not a sprint. It's simply movement. It's a continual progression toward God and away from our flesh. We never arrive, and we never get it all perfect. That's the point!

CHAPTER 5

PHYSICAL FITNESS

I took the love language test, and mine is physical discipline (cue cheesy grin).

WHAT SEEMED LIKE a long season of procrastination turned out to be God's clarification. For years, I've felt this prompting (thanks, Holy Spirit) to write this book. At the time, it made sense to write a book that synced the importance of spiritual fitness with nutrition and exercise. I thought this book would target people who wanted to get physically *fitter*, and they'd be pleasantly surprised to find a few devotional-worthy sentiments too. But in the years of putting off writing, I've dug my heels in deeper to stay grounded in my faith.

God has used this time to reveal to me that this book is not supposed to be a self-improvement book full of healthy recipes and workouts. You can scroll through my Instagram profile to see plenty of resources like that because I think they *are* important. However, God has made it clear. Fitness was never going to be the main purpose of my testimony. It's now just a chapter, pun intended.

Why is it important to be fit?

In Luke 12:42–46, Jesus speaks on what makes a good steward. He implies that a faithful servant and steward is one who is found doing what the Master has asked. For us, we are to manage our gifts, have dominion over the earth, and be fruitful. How we treat our body is a direct reflection of how we treat God's gift. We're to be good stewards of the things of this earth. I believe our body, flesh, and blood belong to God. I'm responsible for how I take care of things (including this body, my health, and my legacy), and I will answer for it at the end of time.

Fitness isn't just important to God. It's important to society. Take a scroll through socials, and you'll be inundated with different descriptions of fitness. You might have found one person's level of fitness inspiring or maybe intimidating. Some say to accept wherever you are as naturally fit. Others say to never quit pursuing improvement. I'd say both are getting close to what God desires for us. To understand a holy pursuit of fitness, we have to value what God says about our bodies and health.

It's true He desires us to prosper and live abundant lives. It's true He brings healing and life. It's true He asks us to be good stewards of all our gifts, including the temple of the Holy Spirit, our body. It's true He calls it good to buffet your body like a boxer but to focus on the disciplines of the heart. All these truths indicate to me that God values our fitness when our motivations are holy. The problems once again are rooted in the foundation of your heart.

Fitness should be a form of worship. Actually, it's always worship. The question is whether our activity is worshiping ourselves or God. When we're motivated only by aesthetics and appearance, we fuel our pride; we are not worshiping God with our fitness. When our physical activities are an outpouring of praise to God, we are doing it right. The ways we exercise are meant to be tactical ways we steward the gifts of health, strength, focus, and perseverance. These are all gifts given to us from God, meant for us to use for His glory, not ours.

What does it mean to be *fit*?

Okay, so we know there are a thousand different definitions of fitness, but we can probably agree that whatever *fit* looks like is subjective. And it's personal.

**Let's redefine *fit* to mean functioning
optimally and growing in potential.**

This is a subjective quality, which eliminates our tendency to compare our own fitness levels to others'.

**Let's redefine *unfit* to mean underperforming and
not utilizing our bodies to grow in potential.**

As a coach, I often assess clients as either conditioned or deconditioned. A conditioned client is someone who can handle pain and push through it. A deconditioned client is someone who has not been through the fire yet. Whew! There's a whole sermon in that concept by itself!

For the sake of this book, and the ideas I'll present regarding physical fitness, it's important for you to consider how conditioned you are in every area of wellness. Questions you can ask yourself include the following:

- *How much experience do you have in this area?*
- *How long have you been intentional to pursue this discipline?*
- *How important is this discipline to you?*
- *What could you use to prove its importance to you?*
- *Recall any specific seasons or moments where you practiced conditioning in this area.*

Maybe you're catching on already, but if not, I hope you can see how the ways I'm approaching physical fitness are very similar to the ways we assess our spiritual fitness. That's precisely why I love incorporating both. We learn about ourselves when we apply pressure. I've learned that's also why life as a Christian is never easy. God wouldn't have us not learning anything. We need to be conditioned so we can be the encouragers to those who are deconditioned.

To be fit means to have evidence that your faith has been tested, and you've come out faithful. Physically, it means you've trained your body to handle pressure and pain. When you're physically fit, you often have less health problems and sickness. At the same time, you often have greater functionality and defense against attacks on your health. To be fit, you have some sort of strategy in place to maintain your wellness.

It's essential we understand that physical disciplines are tactics we implement to train our bodies and in turn train our minds. When we put pressure on our bodies to persevere through pain, we make choices in our minds to either push harder or give up. This will affect your faith. You either learn to become more faithful by choice and through practice, or you don't. You either keep doing the right things or you don't.

To be unfit should be a personal assessment as well. For some, it may mean not doing what you know you should or could be doing, or maybe what you know you're capable of doing to be healthier. Other versions of *unfit* could mean overweight, deconditioned, or symptomatic of an unhealthy condition or illness. Whatever category of *unfit* you fall into, it's important to see it as a starting place and not a final destination, as well as a subjective value dependent on one's individual journey.

For example, I might see myself as less fit during pregnancy compared to years before my pregnancy, but that determination is only relative to my journey, not someone else's. I also may see myself as unfit if I were to suddenly stop performing all the physical disciplines and disregard the strategies I have in place to keep me well, even if I don't see any symptoms of these choices at first. When we become both aware and honest about our personal fitness, we can implement the discipline necessary to grow.

> Be diligent in these matters; give yourself wholly
> to them, so that everyone may see your progress.
> (1 Timothy 4:15)

So much of what I've learned about my spiritual fitness has been learned through my assessment of my physical fitness. As I've tried to implement the discipline necessary to achieve certain standards of physical wellness, I've realized how I needed to grow mentally, emotionally, and spiritually to be able to make those gains. Just like I must be willing to endure a little more discomfort to achieve a new top speed on the treadmill, I also must be willing to endure a little more discomfort in the other areas of wellness to level up.

Physical exercise is a great starting place.

The discipline required to maintain a physical fitness routine teaches you how to maintain consistency despite the way you feel. Physical fitness is probably the most black-and-white, simplest form of establishing a habit of discipline. You either do it or you don't. It's measurable; it's quantifiable. Even if you're not working out at your highest optimal function, you've either made the choice to work out or not. And that, my friends, is the first step to overall fitness. Nike must have been onto something when they said, "Just do it."

There are enough studies, articles, and influencers out now reminding us of the importance of exercise, and it's probably no surprise to hear it from me. Exercise is proven to increase energy and improve hormonal health and sexual libido while also decreasing stress. People who work out are more likely to be what studies call *high achievers*. And if you work out earlier in the day, you tend to get more things done. I can definitely attest to that one!

So if exercise is so important (and simple in concept), why doesn't everyone do it?

It's safe to say most of us are busy, tired, and stressed. I, myself, find it hard to not respond to the casual "How are you?" questions with, "Tired!" We live in a world that glorifies busyness and scoffs at rest unless it's drinking or eating, and maybe the occasional *self-care* routine. When we operate in a stressed state, we are less likely to find a consistent source of motivation to expend more energy. The funny fact is that exercise can actually energize you, even while you burn energy. Most people in my experience don't exercise consistently enough or for a long enough duration to arrive at that energizing place. We have to be willing to implement the activity out of discipline and obedience before we start to feel any pleasure.

Many people are also resistant to exercise because of the promises they hear made to them from companies looking to profit on the desire to receive a bigger payoff than the investment. Many of us, myself included, have fallen prey to the idea that there's an easy way to achieve the results we want. There's a pill, a diet, a powder, a juice, a tea, a specific workout guide, a prayer, a plan, etc., whatever is going to procrastinate me and distract me from doing what I know I should be doing. This is just that—a distraction from the disciplines we should be implementing that require reflection and readjustment from season to season.

I've also found that many people are simply comfortable at the fitness level at which they are. We might describe this type of person as complacent. It's quite easy to be complacent today because society encourages us to accept everyone wherever they are and whoever they are, regardless of the standard. While I agree with the truth that God accepts us all just as we are and that we should accept each other in the same way, I have to add that God does not intend us to stay that way!

On a more practical level, many of us know we need to exercise and try to exercise, but the abundance of information and variety of strategies is overwhelming. Rather than choosing something, anything, we don't choose anything at all, and we don't begin.

Stepping into parenthood and into seasons of blurry, interrupted days, I had to come to an understanding that my perceived ideal way to work out was just not going to be doable anymore. I've learned that there is no *perfect* way to work out. True wellness is about doing something with what you have, rather than waiting for the stars to align and having flawless discipline. Consistency outweighs perfection every time. Consistency with correction leads to improved discipline and wellness.

What kind of exercise is best? (We still all want to know.)

Like I mentioned earlier, any exercise is better than no exercise. I'm sad to say that I've seen too much hating on specific workouts and not enough love for people just getting out there and moving. Even intrinsically, we convince ourselves that we can't exercise because we don't know which exercise(s) to do. Or it's too expensive and takes too much time or we have no childcare.

What you prefer to do might not be best for you in your current season. Once again, I've had to amend my preferences to allow for what I can consistently achieve. During this season, I can consistently work out at home because childcare is not available. I've collected equipment and varied my workouts using these things. I also push my kids in a stroller outside (not because I love the additional weight and stress of toting two, soon-to-be three kids), but because I can do this at no financial cost, and it fits within my family's schedule.

Whatever you do, you should enjoy it. I've met people who tell me they *hate* to work out. Whatever they experienced must not be the right exercise for them. You can dance, swim, rollerblade, cycle, lift, run, jog, or walk. Sometimes, it's not the exercise that's wrong, but it's the environment. What I've loved about group fitness is the atmosphere available that encourages and equips. When you work out with a group of like-minded people, you tend to find it socially and personally rewarding. The effects of accountability help you stay consistently disciplined and corrected to grow in both knowledge and fitness.

I'm physically fittest when I have variety in my workouts. My clients and colleagues agree they are their best selves when their fitness routine involves multiple strategies. And if you're going to do anything for the rest of your life, you better learn to love it and not get tired of it.

If you've never exercised, start with cardio.

Typically, I start out with clients who have little to no experience maintaining an exercise routine with a simple movement. To exhaust your body and rebuild (which is key to growth), you have to have a baseline of fitness. Plus, cardio gives your body and mind the opportunity to work in sync enough that you can *check out* of stress. It's important for one to experience the mental and emotional benefits of exercise, especially while introducing this new discipline.

Cardio is also the most convenient form of exercise since it usually involves little to no equipment and can be assessed with a heart rate monitor or, after the experience, via perceived exertion.

If you need to shape up, lift some weights.

Anyone can read about the benefits to your bone density and skeletal health that lifting weights provides. Aside from those obvious benefits, I think it's especially important because it's the only way to restructure and reshape your body.

Before I started lifting weights, I was convinced I'd never have the definition in my arms I wanted. I thought that genetically, that just wasn't going to happen in my body. The magic of weight lifting is that you can shape your body accordingly. Lifting weights specifies muscular activity so that you can focus on any particular muscle(s) without fatiguing others. This is so helpful when you work out regularly because it prevents overtraining.

Figure out how to combine strength and cardio.

Any combination of cardio and strength is probably my favorite way to work out because it's usually the most intense and most efficient (two of my favorite words). High-intensity interval training (HIIT) is a version of combination work because any time your heart rate is reaching above 75 percent of your maximum heart rate, you're fatiguing your muscles of glycogen as you do during strength training.

Embrace the season of physical fitness you're in and move forward in it.

Life comes in seasons. There are times when I was spending hours working out at the gym and various studios, and I loved it. And then there have been seasons when I'm fighting to get in a twenty-minute workout and trying to make the most of it. I have to conclude that consistency in the discipline of physical exercise is more important than what it looks like.

There may be a season when you take up running and maybe competing in races. There may be a season when you prefer Zumba classes and hot yoga. You may go through a bulk phase, where you do less cardio and spend more time hitting personal records on your lifts. There's no one-size-fits-all type of fitness, and that goes for each person's body every day of their life.

The fittest people I know are the ones who try new things, who go outside their comfort zone to do the things they don't know much about, and who keep their bodies in constant surprise. And that's why it's important to combine your physical fitness goals with all your other wellness goals mentioned in this book.

Before kids, I lifted heavy and spent most of my cardio time on a StairMaster. I taught kickboxing and cycling classes, and I took class at Orangetheory Fitness. After my first child was born, I took up running outdoors again because it was a convenient form of exercise that didn't require child care and took up less of my time. It was a way for me to bond with my son over his first year, introducing him to nature and all the climates Texas generously provides. As I'm now on my third child, I still practice this habit of pushing a stroller outdoors. Running while pushing a double stroller is a whole new workout. Some days, I'd much prefer to be inside the A/C and watching a monitor on my cardio machine, but for the most part, this is what I can consistently do with my children in tow. Therefore, it's what works to maintain my physical discipline in this season of life.

Do you eat to live or live to eat?

Exercise is usually my first step in coaching clients, but nutrition comes shortly after, if not right alongside it. Nutrition involves what you feed your body. Much like exercise, the excessive amount of information available can make anyone turn a blind eye to knowledge and just eat what they feel like eating. This is the problem I've encountered the most when it comes to the clients who approach me for help. Most people aren't without knowledge, but they're suffocating in it. Most are confused about what works for their personal needs.

I approach nutrition the same way I do fitness. Some nutritional guidelines are more or less effective depending on your season of life. Part of the journey is exploring food and discovering what works for you today while accepting that you may have to explore and discover something new later.

Regardless, you have to commit to something and stick with it. Whether you find out the approach is not best for your personal lifestyle or you find out it's exactly what you need to do, you have to do something consistently. This brings me to a very strong point I'd like to make when it comes to fueling your body: diet with caution.

There are problems with dieting or following *meal plans* that stay the same for long periods. First, your body gets the same limited nutrition, which prevents your body from getting new sources of vitamins, minerals, and other benefits of having variety in your food. Second, and more importantly, a diet becomes a crutch so that when you transition out of a diet, you don't know how to handle freedom with food. The restriction that diets typically include is like having helicopter parents who never let you do anything on your own, too many rules leading to a rebellion.

When I competed in bodybuilding shows, diets were extreme and essential. Combined with my already messed-up mental state of trying to control my food and restrictive eating, I found myself idolizing the occasional *treat meals*. I glorified food. This was an extreme case, and one that sometimes we have to experience, so we understand how to grow and improve our psyche around food.

Yet what I've learned from coaching myself and others is that for the average person who wants to be fit, look and feel good, and have a stellar operating system from the inside out, it's best to focus on eating habits. How can you correct your eating habits as if you were going to adjust them to last for a lifetime, not just for thirty days? As a caveat, it might be beneficial to implement some restrictions at first but always as a strategy that leads to gaining more freedom with food.

Here are five fundamentals of nutrition:

1. Intuitive eating versus dieting

This is a practice I make almost all my clients go through for at least a week. By the time most people ask for help with their nutrition, they've experienced what I call a *diet mentality*. When you restrict or reward yourself regarding food, you give food power over you. So much of the strength we can pursue involves taking ownership of our thoughts, feelings, and actions, so any power given to something as daft as food is just nonsense. We must get away from this mentality and start thinking of food as a fuel source, as a healing source, and as a means to growth.

Diets are a merry-go-round of emotional eating. You engage your willpower to stick to a diet and then reward yourself when you feel like you've accomplished something. As soon as that happens, you feel bad, and you restrict yourself. This type of restriction is a punishment, not a discipline. Because it's a punishment, the repercussions, however long this goes for, are not supporting long-term nutrition goals. This is not healthy. Intuitive eating goes hand in hand with the habits of intrinsic motivation and discipline. This is why establishing value to discipline in general and from a holistic viewpoint is so important.

I often have clients make notes about all their food choices for at least three days. This forces the client to be more mindful of what they're eating and helps them understand why they're making the choice they are. Maybe they've chosen this snack because they've been choosing it for years, eating it at the same time of day. Or maybe they discover they make choices based on the choices of others. Take as much time as you need to get this intuitive eating thing down. This part is foundational to any of the next steps; otherwise, it will always feel restrictive and like a diet. You must learn to be in charge of your choices. Surround yourself with people who will keep you accountable (a balance between challenging you and supporting you). Your friends should never shame you for ordering something *healthy*, or not partaking in alcohol.

2.   Get in your greens.

On a more practical level, eat more vegetables than you feel like eating. Once again, our busy lives are to blame for this one. Eating more veggies requires more planning, shopping, preparing, etc. Aside from that, most people complain that they just don't like certain foods. If we're still struggling with that side of things, you might ask yourself if you're willing to do what's uncomfortable now to gain freedom forever.

Vegetables are the safest way to fuel your body with the nutrients it needs. Over time, you begin to *want* to eat vegetables. They provide more vitamins, antioxidants, and minerals than other foods, as well as offer a nutrient-dense yet calorically weak foundation for your diet, giving you more room to play with other foods.

If you're really struggling with eating veggies because they cause discomfort in the gut (gas, bloating, etc.), then start out eating them slightly cooked instead of raw. Also try taking some digestive enzymes before eating to prepare your body to break down the fibrous materials.

3.   Water makes the world go round.

When I refer to nutrition, I'd be remiss to not include hydration. This is probably the simplest yet most common area people fail. Most of us probably walk around slightly dehydrated most of our life. So many symptoms of discomfort and lack of progress can be improved by drinking more water.

The average person should try to drink around 100 ounces of water per day. The last thing I want this book to do is to give you a legalistic strategy to success, but that quantity is a decent yet daunting average for most people. Track how much water you drink on average over a couple of days, and add increments of 20 ounces until you habitually reach 100 ounces per day. The idea is that most people are walking around slightly dehydrated, which immediately places the body in a state of underperformance. It also makes the body vulnerable to illness and fatigue. I recommend drinking most of your water in between meals so that you don't disrupt digestion.

4. *Figure out what fuels you and focus on it.*

Food is way more than just fuel, but as far as nutrition goes, that's what it is. Food may not be exactly like medicine, but it can both amplify your immune system or adversely affect your health. I like coaching clients on this concept of food as fuel because it typically directly confronts our idolized perception of food.

For many of us, food is a comfort that has become a coping mechanism. It's a temporary high or sometimes, a mindless, mechanical thing we do when we're stressed. Understanding what your body needs and when it needs it is foundational to fixing all your health issues. For most of us, in America, we have access to endless options, so learning how to regulate how much food to eat is a good starting point.

From there, we address the concept of real food versus bioengineered food. Coming back to what God provided through Creation gives us a good umbrella of food choices. Simply put, these are foods that can be named by single words (i.e., apple, avocado, egg). This would push options that have artificial ingredients down to the bottom of the list. Again, this doesn't mean we can't consume them, but we learn that they provide very little fuel, if any at all.

Ideally, I strive to personally eat all macronutrients (protein, fat, and carbohydrates), and I desire my clients to reach this freedom as well. There are reasons we would emphasize one macronutrient more than others, but all are good.

Generally speaking, protein is the macronutrient on which I make sure my clients are focused. Once this is in check, we can manipulate how much fat and carbohydrates someone can eat, depending on their health history and goals. Someone who has hormonal issues may need to focus on eating more nutrient-dense fats and less carbohydrates, while someone who is trying to build muscle may need to focus on eating less food from fat and more from readily digestible carbohydrates. The actual breakdown of macronutrients and calories is less important though, than ensuring the source of these macros is healthy.

For protein, pick meat, eggs, and dairy. When you eat meat, opt for organic poultry, grass-fed beef, and wild-caught seafood because they're the most nutritionally dense options. The organic, grass-fed, and wild-caught variations are important because these products are often more regulated in our food industry than the others and less likely to contain nonfood elements. Regulation in the food industry is unfortunately not as reliable as we would hope or think, so we should take responsibility to know as well as we can what kind of protein we are putting into our bodies.

For fats, focus on grass-fed butter, bacon grease, coconut, avocado, and extra virgin olive oil. These fats feed your body the fuel it needs to produce healthy hormone functions. When your hormones are functioning optimally, your body will respond appropriately to stress, as well as alert you when you're either full or hungry. Healthy hormones support a healthy metabolism, which is the furnace of burning fat as energy. As important as it is to consume healthy fats, it's equally as important to avoid rancid and trans fats, which will wreak havoc on your hormones and metabolism. Examples include seed oils like palm, cottonseed, soybean, and anything hydrogenated. These oils have typically undergone processing that when ingested will disrupt normal hormonal function, causing your metabolism to slow down, as well as cause gut inflammation, which affects your hormones and metabolisms too.

For carbohydrates, keep vegetables and fruit as the most copious choices. Once again, vegetables and fruits are less processed foods and offer more nutritional benefits like vitamins and antioxidants. This doesn't mean other carbohydrates are bad. It's about identifying what the role of the food is. A big bowl of oats might replenish your body's glycogen stores after a few days of fasting or enduring lots of physical stress. Like the other macronutrients, you have to avoid the kinds of carbohydrates that have been processed to include artificial ingredients. For example, a tortilla may have wheat in it, which is not awful, but it also has binders, sweeteners, and fillers, that are.

5. *Cut the crap.*

Too many people are stuffing kale and celery into their blenders and are still discouraged from not seeing results. Most times, it's because they're not removing the other junk food they're still eating. This principle really has to occur in unison with the intuitive eating principle. If you simply detox or throw out all the junk, or make vows to "never eat this or that," you might be stepping into that restriction zone again. We must understand that cleaning the junk out of our kitchens is a strategy to set us up to begin afresh. It's similar to the principle involved in a situation where someone who wanted to stop drinking alcohol would get rid of all the alcohol in their house. The hope is that one day, they can be around alcohol or even partake in a casual drink without it enslaving them like it used to.

I don't like to put labels like *bad* or *good* on foods, but there are foods that are higher quality and lower quality. There are also foods that are going to fuel your body better for the goals you have in mind. This part of the journey toward physical wellness is similar to the spiritual discipline of fasting. It's saying no for now, not forever. This is why it's important to have a plan in place. To be mindful is to use discipline.

Purge your pantry of foods that are causing bloating and other gut issues. Do an overhaul of your kitchen so that there's nothing in-house that will derail your nutrition. This is so simple yet so essential to maintaining your discipline with food. And many times, this is a game changer to success because it goes against what you want, and it might even feel a bit restrictive. But we do so because we are disciplined, not because we are punishing ourselves. I often remind clients that we're not telling ourselves no forever, just for now.

I also encourage my clients to eliminate these foods from their weekly shopping list. Once again, it's not that these are never allowed to enter our bodies, but it should not be a part of our normal daily nutrition.

- processed gluten (cereals, premade sauces, etc.)
- additives (give a list of bad ingredients)

- trans fats
- processed sugar (basically any sugar that doesn't occur naturally, and even natural sugar should be very small)
- added sugar

You have to make the choice to implement holistic discipline as a family choice.

Early on in my marriage, nutrition was a topic of conflict. Micah had a very different view of it than me. We both had to learn and grow together. We both now agree on wellness as a priority for our family, and we both try to support each other in the strategies we have in place. This doesn't mean we eat the same meal for every meal every day. Micah's food looks different than mine, and depending on whether I'm pregnant or training for something, our grocery list can look vastly different. The point is not that we are the same, but that our visions are the same. We are unified. We support each other.

With kids involved in our family now, we are learning how to implement these disciplines for kids too. We are also passionate about teaching our kids these same lessons, as difficult as it is in the world of chicken nuggets and goldfish in which we live. We've decided that to live differently is worth it. And it's also worth it to have a constant student mindset, one in which we are continually learning, adjusting, and growing, and letting our children participate.

Other tips for eating smarter are as follows:

- Plan more (make a list of groceries and for meals).
- Shop more often and shop smarter (perimeter of the store first).
- Learn to cook (start simply).
- Invest in some decent cooking utensils and serving ware.

Do you not know that you are God's temple and that God's Spirit dwells in you? If anyone destroys God's temple, God will destroy him. For

God's temple is holy, and you are that temple. (1
Corinthians 3:16–17)

Physical fitness is not rocket science; it's actually very simple. Sometimes, the simplest of things are the hardest to accomplish. It's uncomfortable, and we live in a world that idolizes comfort. Nobody else can be fit for you. No pill, no workout, no trainer, no pair of shoes, no diet, no other thing can do it for you.

Once you value physical fitness and perceive it as a command-ment from God Himself, it changes everything. At the same time, once you understand how the journey to physical wellness parallels the journey to spiritual fitness, the idea of success becomes much more attainable and rewarding.

CHAPTER 6

MENTAL FITNESS

Where the mind goes, the man follows.

—Joyce Meyer

MY PERSONAL JOURNEY to become mentally strong did not intentionally start until I understood the value of personal growth. I didn't value personal growth until I started trying to make improvements to my physical health. The challenges I faced while enduring physical pain and trying things that exposed my weakness forced me to face the weaknesses in my mind. For me to say yes to another rep, a heavier weight load, or a faster speed, I had to choose to embrace the pain. That takes mental strength!

How do you evaluate your mental fitness?

Have you ever stopped to think about what you've been thinking about lately? As funny as that sounds, it's imperative to our wellness that we become acutely aware of our thought patterns and self-talk.

Until I started following someone else's fitness program and training regimen planned for me, I had never really pushed myself physically. Sure, there were things I did that included faith over fear like tumbling and stunts (in cheerleading) and some intense cardio sessions on the treadmill. But for the most part, I was comfortable with being comfortable.

When I committed to training for a bodybuilding competition, I signed up for lifting lots of heavy weights. I remember sitting on this crazy contraption called a leg press for the first time. After twenty seconds, I found myself trying to suck the tears back into my eyeballs because I was so frustrated with my weakness and obvious lack of physical ability. I remember questioning whether or not to just get up and go to the cardio section. I contemplated telling my trainer that I'd made a mistake; this was not going to work. I'm pretty sure the biggest motivation at the time for me was the fear of being embarrassed over quitting so early on, but whatever it was that kept me on that leg press worked. I pushed through the tears with my shaky legs and somehow managed to finish my first *leg day*. I took it one day at a time for many months on end, trying to improve just a little bit every chance I got. I realized that if I wanted to get physically stronger, I needed to get mentally stronger.

The intense sessions on the StairMaster provided an opportunity for me to distract myself for long periods with my phone. I remember getting severely bored with my music after a couple of weeks, so I started watching shows. Then I remember getting bored with shows (and the absolute nonsense I was shoving into my brain for the allotment of time), so I switched to listening to sermons from church. Then I moved to YouTube videos and podcasts. I used the time I was physically training my body to grow to also mentally train my mind to grow. I fed my mind the fuel it needed to make the gains.

As I learned about the power of words and thoughts by listening and reading content from healthy, spiritual leaders, I gained valuable personal intel. I learned I needed to take inventory of my habitual patterns of thinking. Below are some examples of toxic thought patterns which I had habitually gleaned; they're written in ways I talked to myself, especially amid pain or conflict.

- If you can't excel at it, quit before you fail at it.
- Others are judging you.

- If you're not immediately good at it, then you will never be good at it, and it's a waste of time.
- You will never be as good as you want to be, and you'll definitely not ever be as good as *her*.
- This can't be what God has for you or planned for you because of all the pain involved.
- You're going to be weak forever; you're not good enough to improve.
- No one will ever love you the way you are, so you might as well get used to this.

These are just a sample of some of the toxic thoughts God revealed to me after I became aware of the weaknesses in my mind. Dealing with the perseverance of physical discipline led me to an awareness of the mental discipline necessary to grow stronger from the inside out.

If you've never taken an inventory of your thoughts, I'd recommend taking a few days and being mindful of it. One approach is to try to be silent for a couple of days and only write down your thoughts. The other is to simply pause after thinking to yourself. Make a chart of the positive thoughts you think and the negative thoughts you think. You can even mark the ideas you put words to and separate them from the ones that you keep locked away.

We have to get to a point where we're willing, to be honest with ourselves if we truly want to grow. We have to move from a state of being inspired to a state of being intentional if we want to see the results of habitual discipline.

Have you talked to yourself lately?

Self-talk is a simple way of describing the conversations you have in your mind but never say out loud (or around others). If you've ever tried on an outfit and thought, "Gah, I'm so fat." That's an example of self-talk.

Habitual self-talk is taking a thought to the next level: entertaining it and playing with it. Negative self-talk is dangerous because it creates a pattern of thinking. You're literally training your brain into believing what you're thinking by repeating the same thoughts over and over again.

We can choose to train our brains to believe either positive or negative things about ourselves. Even those who speak the fewest words have conversations in their minds. It's truly the beginning of all habits, patterns, and actions, whether we want to stay the same or change.

When we become aware of the power of our thoughts, and even more so, our habitual thought patterns, we can see the consistency (or inconsistencies) between who people say we are and who *we* say we are. When we're aware of the dangerous ground bred in our thoughts, we can sometimes fall into an even more dangerous trap of living divided. This happens when someone has a difference between their self-talk and the evidence exhibited in his or her actions.

> We demolish arguments and every pretension
> that sets itself up against the knowledge of God,
> and we take captive every thought to make it
> obedient to Christ. (2 Corinthians 10:5)

There's a transition period in personal growth when we become aware of our negative thoughts, and therefore, we try to speak more positively about ourselves and those around us. Speaking words out loud is another strategy to train our brains. We hear those words, and they start to replace our thoughts. This occurrence is totally normal and necessary to recreate habits of positive thinking. This is different than when our actions and expressions directly contradict our beliefs. It's normal to still have negative thoughts, but pause to take inventory of them before replacing them in our minds with a godly truth. That's healing. We want to avoid saying one thing and thinking another without replacing the thought in our self-talk. When we replace lies with truth, we change what we believe, and that's the key to true healing from toxic thought patterns.

Keep in mind another mental snare the evil will leave for you is the fear of being a hypocrite. While you're busy trying to better yourself, the enemy will often try to trip you up by reminding you of how unqualified you are. Thoughts and/or past memories will haunt you. The truth is that *this* is where the battle is won or lost. What will you believe about yourself?

Another trap to beware of is when you remove authenticity from the equation. When someone talks a big game about themselves, but they're really struggling with self-hate and doubt and never honest with anyone else about it, that's an example of living divided. All that person's actions begin to live as lies. That's when we're walking on dangerous ground. That's why seeking God's truth, coming back to your *why*, and having a circle of accountability are all essential parts of personal growth and getting stronger from the inside out.

Do you have thoughts you meditate on?

> My son, be attentive to my words; incline your ear to my sayings. Let them not escape from your sight; keep them within your heart. For they are life to those who find them, and healing to all their flesh. (Proverbs 4:20–22)

Ten years ago, I would have told you meditation is only something they do in yoga classes or in the Eastern world. Yet as I've studied scripture and applied godly principles, I realize that we all meditate on thoughts, whether we mean to or not. God asks us to meditate on His Word, but do we really do that?

The thoughts we have most often are the ones on which we meditate. Like a broken record on repeat, these are the thoughts that pop up again and again, without us really trying to think about them. They are the ones making the biggest impact on our actions and emotions. You can think yourself stressed. You can also think yourself into feeling calm and at peace.

Changing these meditations is how we both practice and improve our mental strength. Once again, it requires mindfulness, intentionality, and discipline. We need to practice it on good days and remind ourselves to do it even on bad days. We may do it more easily on good days, but it's the bad days that these mental habits will work for us or against us.

How do you meditate or change your thoughts?

There were times I pleaded to God and even to others in conflict, "I can't change the way I feel." I realize now that I can actually change the way I feel when I change the way I think. Yes, I believe that I still experience emotions that are very real in my physiology, but I believe that the truth of God's Word is much more powerful than my feelings.

I've found that reading scripture and then writing it down in my own words helps me to remember it later. When I think about the principle in play in the scripture and how it applies to me personally, I'm personalizing God's Word. I'm creating a new thought pattern that I can rehearse throughout the day. This doesn't guarantee that I won't have negative thoughts that pop into my mind, but I'm now more likely to contrast that bad thought with this new, good thought, and choose to believe the good one over the bad.

A key consideration when trying to apply these changes to our thought patterns is to remember that our thoughts do not have to be supported by our feelings. There are many (maybe even most) times that I choose to believe what God says about me even when I don't feel it. I can choose to believe that I'm more than a conqueror (Romans 8:37) when I feel like a failure. I can choose to believe that God is faithful (1 Corinthians 1:9) when I'm disappointed. I can choose to believe that God loves me (Zephaniah 3:17) when others do not. And in all these things, I can rehearse these thoughts over and over again until the lies are silenced.

I mentioned a sample of toxic thought patterns I battled when I first began my journey to intentional personal growth. I'd be remiss to not mention that I still have toxic thoughts I battle. They are less habitual, and I wouldn't say they are strongholds in my mind like they used to be. But they are negative thoughts that I must overcome by intentionally meditating on God's truth. I'm learning that the journey to wellness is never-ending. That's just it; it's a journey!

Some of the thoughts that introduce lies to me mentally and try to steal my confidence in God's purposes for me would include the following.

- *You have nothing valuable to offer anyone.*
- *Anything you think you know or can do, someone else can do better.*
- *You've worked so hard, and you still have nothing to show for it.*
- *You are being prideful and conceited to think that anyone would need you or want you.*

I mention these to emphasize that all who claim to follow Jesus are human fleshly beings trying to listen and obey. We choose who we worship, who we obey, and which thoughts control our actions. Yes, these thoughts both distract and frustrate me. However, they do so less and less as I practice fighting the battle in my mind to replace lies with truth. Every time I choose to think intentionally and focus on what God says instead of what I think or feel, I strengthen my faith and conviction in who He is. When I strengthen my awareness of who He is, I discover who I really am.

Finding God through salvation is not the end-all destination. We find God, and we are filled with His Spirit, so we can get healthier. We can then engage in a powerful, enjoyable journey from that point forward. We do not arrive at our endpoint until we meet Him face to face. Until then we march forward, getting stronger from the inside out.

CHAPTER 7

EMOTIONAL FITNESS

Feelings aren't bad, but they're not God.

EARLY ON IN marriage, I realized I am a deeply sensitive feeler. I also realized my husband is not. It's taken me years to determine that one way is not better than the other. One way is not more righteous nor more godly. In fact, men and women and our personality differences are both necessary to represent the fullness of godly expression in marriage and family.

I've alluded to this concept earlier when I mentioned that we live in a culture that justifies action based on emotion. "I do what I want," or "I'm not feeling it," are commonly held beliefs by today's generation. We accept people for how they feel, and to a fault, we make allowances for apathy, immorality, and deviance from biblical principles. However, I don't want to dismiss the importance of feelings.

God gave humanity the ability to feel, to experience emotion. The Bible mentions Jesus being moved with compassion many times. Paul warned the church in his writing to not grieve the Holy Spirit. We can conclude that God Himself throughout the Bible experienced emotions like anger, sadness, grief, joy, and pleasure. Since we are made in His image, we are to experience these emotions as well. I have to believe that this is because there's a purpose to our feelings.

Just like any other innate part of humanity, what's meant to be a blessing to us, to draw us closer into intimacy with God can also reel us away from Him. For years, I struggled with getting so caught up in the way I felt, I lost sense of reality. It would take hours if not days for me to recover from a deeply felt feeling. This caused tension in my relationships because even though I was desperately trying to forgive or *get over it*, I felt powerless in my feelings. And they were so strong!

Arguments with my husband would go into the early morning hours. My deep emotions contrasted with his feelings. We felt divided. I would only feel more and more isolated, as I felt completely misunderstood and at times, just crazy.

I was constantly offended.

Offense positions you to fight battles you were never meant to fight, nor will you ever truly win. That's what was happening to me. I was constantly offended (and I still can be). Being angry is not bad. But we are to only use holy emotions that help us fight for what is important to God. If we're busy fighting battles we have no business fighting, then we'll be too exhausted to fight the battles God sets us up in.

Over the years, as I've sought the Lord, especially using my deep emotions, I've learned so much. God created me to experience feelings deeply. They're not bad. I'm not wrong. God has given me the gift to feel things deeper, and like all God-given gifts, it's something to be used for His glory and my good. I have to grow in my knowledge of God and specifically, the Holy Spirit, as He operates in me every day. If I'm to steward the gift to draw deeper into a relationship with God and others, then I must be emotionally healthy.

If thoughts can lead to feelings, and feelings can emphasize thoughts, which thoughts do you want to feed?

As someone who experiences deep emotion, even in the most menial tasks, I find that I can get lost in the thoughts surrounding my feelings. As I mentioned in the previous chapter, thoughts can lead to feelings. However, feelings can lead to thoughts too. If I'm not careful, a deeply experienced feeling can drive me to arrive at a lie. At the very least, I can experience emotions so deep that I arrive at unrealistic expectations which only lead to disappointment.

Just like the other disciplines, we must periodically assess our emotional fitness. For some, this may be the first time they've ever stopped to ask themselves how they're feeling. For others, this may be something you already practice regularly. Regardless, the best way to approach it is to be intentional with the reflective process.

For those who tend to be less emotional and more logical, like my husband, it may be wise to seek counsel in this area to determine which emotions others notice you expressing. Once again, humility is essential here. One has to be willing to hear the hard truth and possibly face painful remarks as well as be open to understanding something of which you were once unaware. All people, even the toughest ones, express emotions. If you think you don't, you're most likely unaware they're showing. And the dangerous part is that the emotions you're really feeling may be surfacing as something else. If we want others to truly know us, which is an integral desire God has given us all, then we must be willing to get honest with ourselves and others.

For example, many times in conversation, I'll suggest my husband may be angry, for that's the emotion he's expressing. He often corrects me that he's frustrated with something. And if we dig deeper, we conclude he's either feeling frustrated with himself or others because he had an unmet expectation. When we have unmet expectations, we can often feel helpless or hopeless. If we've tried in our own power to make something happen, and it doesn't, we can feel helpless. When we realize we've emptied our energy only to result in an unmet expectation, we can then feel hopeless. These are specific words that would describe a level of hurt. Many times, people who are hurt may express themselves with anger.

For example, when parenting our children, my husband and I both can often describe ourselves as frustrated, angry, and at our wits' end. Usually, after reflecting on why we feel the way we do, we understand it's because we somehow convinced ourselves that if we did *A*, *B*, and *C*, our children would behave with *D*, *E*, and *F*. We find ourselves hurt over the fact we've done everything in our power to help our children either obey or be successful, and they still fall short. Unfortunately, we're learning that as parents, we can only exert so much influence over our children. We can ensure we've communicated clearly and implemented consequences, but we cannot make our children do anything they don't choose to do. Understanding this truth and learning from experience is truly frustrating!

Here are some questions to assess your emotional fitness:

- Do I know the emotions I'm currently feeling?
- Are my emotions adding to my energy or draining my energy?
- Am I experiencing physical effects caused by emotions?
- Am I successful at maintaining self-control?
- Am I succeeding or failing, and why do I think this?
- How have I rested lately? Do I need more rest?
- How would others describe me or the atmosphere when I'm around?

Another consideration for assessing one's emotional fitness is to evaluate one's emotional intelligence. How much do you understand the power of emotions? Do you have the ability to perceive the emotions exhibited in yourself and others?

Some of us were modeled healthy articulation of feelings, but most of us probably weren't. For example, emotions were always expressed in my childhood home, but no accountability or self-control was really modeled. One could feel what they felt and do whatever they felt like with those feelings with very few consequences to follow. Outbursts and rage were common.

However, in my husband's home, emotions were bottled up, squashed, and swallowed. He grew to believe that any negative emotion was pointless to feel or express. While I see so much strength in my husband after he's learned to exhibit self-control and power over his emotions, he'd agree with me that he's also struggled to even put a word to the way he feels at times. As healthy humans, we must learn to acknowledge our feelings without allowing them to dominate our behavior in an ungodly way. This requires discipline.

What I love about applying the concept of discipline to my emotions is that it reveals what we can control and what we cannot. I may have a feeling that strikes me out of nowhere, that I don't want to feel for too long, and knowing that I can control how the feeling affects me is a powerful thought. I do not have to be a slave to my feelings nor does anyone else.

Like most of this content, I've learned how to apply discipline to my emotional fitness through the practice of discipline in my wellness habits. I've made it clear that discipline and consistency in our habits are two essential pillars of being well. To understand wellness, we also have to understand that overall wellness will be redefined over and over depending on our season of life and level of personal growth. In turn, we find out that there will be seasons of momentum, where we feel unstoppable. And there will be seasons where it feels like a fight to get one inch ahead.

If I haven't convinced you yet to stop and reflect now and again on what you're thinking and how you're feeling, at least consider this. The people you love will be affected by your thoughts and feelings. The atmosphere will change with you in it, whether you realize it or not. God has given us the power to influence for His glory. The question of all questions we should ask ourselves when it comes to emotional fitness is this: Are we or are we not using the power God gives us within our relationship for the good of others and for God's glory?

CHAPTER 8

PATIENCE AND PERSEVERANCE

WE JUST WRAPPED up in the last several chapters how wellness is more than just our physical health. To be well means we are flourishing in our physical fitness, spiritual fitness, mental fitness, and emotional fitness. In each of these areas, we should be growing. We should be getting stronger.

But what about when it's hard to grow? What do we do when we've lost our motivation to keep going and the discipline we've implemented thus far feels fruitless?

Motivation is a feeling. Discipline is a choice.

When we try to change the outside without discipline, the weakness inside prevents us from succeeding. When we are motivated from the inside out, we naturally affect the outside. Motivation is inspired by our emotions, while discipline is practiced despite our emotions.

I've shared this analogy a thousand times with clients. It used to take discipline for me to practice brushing my teeth. Discipline is still heavily required regarding toothbrushing time for my children. If they brushed their teeth when they felt like it, their teeth would look like Cheetos Puffs. One of my jobs as a parent is to equip them with the knowledge and power to be able to discipline themselves to form the habit of dental hygiene. Once the habit's created, they will no longer refuse to brush their teeth or whine about it but will instead eagerly head to the sink and slap some paste on their brush. I've seen this in real life transform in my oldest child.

It may seem silly to relate discipline and dental hygiene, but it's true. It's also fairly simple. Every habit we have or don't have is dependent on discipline. The ability to choose something that defies feelings, paired with consistency, is what makes an attitude or action a habit. It doesn't matter if it's brushing your teeth or working out.

Discipline can create habits, but motivation will not. Feeling motivated is a great feeling, but it often fades. When it fades, you have to rely on the discipline of your soul. And beyond that, you have to rely on the power of the Holy Spirit to work within you. That's why it's so important to consider wellness holistically.

Godly discipline tells me to control what only I can control. Your discipline is only as good as the degree to which you trust God more than yourself. You demonstrate that trust by relinquishing control of anyone or anything else other than your own soul.

Discipline without a God-focused perspective is only willpower.

When taken to the extreme, without submission to God, discipline says you can control it all. It says you're to blame for every failure and also to credit for every success. This type of discipline can equate to the worldly understanding of willpower. It's prevalent among fitness accounts all over social media. It causes shame and blame and can keep us all from journeying forward in God's favorable plan.

Discipline without submission says you can control your marriage, your kids, your home, your body, and your happiness. One who operates with this type of discipline will often take on a martyr mentality that seeks to take care of everyone and everything (yeah, that was me), shortly followed by a victim mentality. Often, you will take on other people's emotions as both your responsibility and a reflection of you. This starts a cycle of service, disappointment, judgment, and self-loathing, and then back to service. Often the service part is done with pure intentions, but sometimes, it's done as penance because you feel bad about judging others or because you're trying to win back other people's favor so you can try to control them again.

Something about having children has forced me to reconcile this part of me. I'm far from completely delivered from so-called control issues, but I'm getting there. It's been a part of my journey. The hard part about relinquishing control as a parent is that there are primary functions a parent keeps that rely on their capacity to control their kids. My husband and I control their home environment, their food, their school, their activities, etc. The older our children get, the less control we will invoke over their lives, with the hopes that the training through which we've brought them will equip them to make righteous choices on their own.

So much of the control we try to take is learned from how our parents treated us as kids. I have tended to model the controlling behavior of my mom, in error, while my brothers tend to model the passive, controllable behaviors of my dad. Either way is not good. When two parties who operate differently like this come together, we become codependent. I've learned that the biggest blessing for me as a wife has been my husband's relentless resistance to me controlling him.

When my inability to control others slaps me in the face, I have to turn to God. He's the only one who can show me how to detach myself from that codependent relationship and return to being fully dependent on God alone. I've had to implement discipline in this area because frankly, I don't often feel motivated to turn to God. I often feel motivated to try to convince someone else why I'm right and how if they'd just listen to me, they'd be better for it.

Sometimes, we have to come face to face with our own failures and disappointments so that we can turn our face to God, who heals, restores, and fills. If this is not part of your journey toward wellness, then I'm sorry to be the bearer of this news, but your journey will plateau long before you reach your potential.

So how do we move from motivation to discipline?

In whichever field we're trying to apply discipline, we must reflect on why we're pursuing whatever it is we're pursuing. If it's physical fitness, why? If it's a new job, why? If it's financial freedom, why? If it's a relationship, why? Our answers reveal our intentions, which will reveal your emotional attachment to the journey.

When we know how we feel about someone or something, we can better prevent ourselves from acting in a way that will cause detriment to our end goals. For example, if my goal is to improve my relationship with my husband, to feel loved and cherished and intimate, I'd ask myself why I want this. I might answer myself with a response that says I no longer want to feel unloved, overlooked, or distant from my spouse. When I claim how I feel now and how I want to feel, I claim control over myself and release my spouse from my control. I also reveal the strategy to get to my goal; I must change the way I feel, the way I think, and the way I act. I can't do this without discipline.

When we don't know our purpose, we get distracted by other people's purposes.

Most understand how comparison steals our joy. Have you ever wondered why? I often wonder why it's so hard to celebrate other people without simultaneously feeling let down. Before comparison steals our joy, it steals our attention.

We begin to emphasize either the successes or failures of others and measure our own worth to theirs. Comparison can be used in godly ways to mature and grow and model. But an unhealthy person can't handle it that way. Typically, comparison leads us to one of two conclusions: we're better or we're worse. If we don't know how to control these feelings and thoughts, they could lead to either pride or shame.

One of the greatest ways to stay disciplined in this area is to think about thankfulness. What fills you with gratitude? We will never be excited to do what it takes to arrive at a better future if we're ungrateful for what we have. However, we gain momentum moving forward when we position ourselves in a place of gratitude.

Often when I'm feeling purposeless or disappointed, I'll think about thankfulness. If it's regarding someone in particular, I'll think about something this person has recently done or said that makes me feel good. I'll celebrate the victories I see in that person (or even myself) and ask God to make me blind to the bad. It's not my job to point out the bad. It's God's. I have to trust Him to do what He says.

How do you get grateful when you feel overlooked, overworked, and overwhelmed?

First, we need to agree that God does not intend for His children to live this way. We are supposed to live as heirs to the King, children of God, with freedom, joy, and peace.

> You make known to me the path of life; in your presence there is fullness of joy; at your right hand are pleasures forevermore. (Psalm 16:11)

When we feel overlooked, it's often because we are too busy looking around. We look at social media. We look at our friends and family. We look to our spouse. We look to our kids. And many times, we look those ways before we look to God. If we look to others to affirm us, we will feel disappointed every time.

Pastor Mike Todd of Transformation Church in Oklahoma has said that when the enemy can't successfully destroy something in your life, he will distract you. We have to understand that being distracted grieves God. He desires our whole heart. Any time we reserve a part of our attention to something or someone above Him, we are practicing idolatry.

We must stay focused on God and reel ourselves in when we feel this overlooked. We must ask the hard questions of why we feel this way. We must practice discipline in the areas of mental and emotional fitness to determine how we got this way. Finally, we must look to the Father. This may mean a night of worship instead of Netflix, an earlier alarm to spend time with God, or a purposeful prayer in the shower.

When we feel overworked, we have to determine why we are working in the first place. In my experience, I've once again fallen into the trap of trying to work to win people. I also try to work to win God's approval. When we understand we already have God's full approval, adoption, and attention, we can stop working for it. It's out of His grace that He chooses to love us first, even if we're not saved and living like heathens (been there, done that).

Many of us may have grown up feeling loved after we did something right. Loving affirmations from friends and family, although righteous, can also teach us that love is to be earned. It's one of the slickest tricks of the enemy. He uses the sweet words of a loving mom, who says, "Aw, great job doing the dishes, baby. I love you so much," to lie to the child. The kid grows up thinking, *I'm loved when I work hard.* It's a narrow path, and it's so hard to navigate.

This is why it's imperative for us to live filled with the spirit of God, alive and speaking to us in personal ways. We need Him to tell us what's dysfunctional and what's not. We need Him to reveal to us why we are the way we are and how to journey forward.

When we feel overwhelmed, it's because we feel hopeless about who we are or what we're doing. It's often because we hold ourselves in a position only God can reign. We put pressure on ourselves to be and do things we were never created to be and do. We may be carrying a cross that isn't ours to carry. Yes, we all have a cross we're created to carry, but if we don't give what rightly belongs to God, to Him, we will feel the weight of it all our days, and we will tire out.

One personal example is the weight of unforgiveness. Through researching and writing this book, the Holy Spirit revealed a new level of forgiveness I was to enter into with my family. He identified certain offenses I was constantly carrying and the bitterness that was growing inside me. Even deeper, He revealed to me the forgiveness I was withholding from myself. If I don't totally forgive myself, and instead try to work my sins off, I get overwhelmed. That's a penance I will never repay. I'm essentially telling Jesus that the work He did on the cross, the payment He already made, isn't enough.

Unforgiveness, resentment, bitterness, or sinful habits will always keep us from experiencing the peace God intends us to have in all seasons of our life. The world tells us peace comes from things, feelings, or people. God desires us to encounter peace by abiding in His presence. Sometimes, our involvement with religion trains us to think we need to be punished for all the bad things we've done, and maybe then we can get a glimpse of peace. However, true peace is not attained by doing anything or having anything. In fact, true peace is often experienced in the midst of pain.

Pain has been the best breeding ground for peace in my life. I suppose that's why fitness is so important to me. The pain involved in training both my body and brain parallels the pain through which I persevere in all other aspects of life. Just like my body gets stronger as I learn to push through pain in a workout, my spirit gets stronger as I learn to lean into God at the most uncomfortable of times. Learning how to access the peace God makes available to me requires me to discipline myself while under the pressures of life.

Discipline means controlling your emotions and sometimes denying your will.

One thing we need to understand is that God makes His peace available to all who submit to Him. We have to believe that to access that gift. Peace is not an atmosphere I can achieve or a feeling I can muster up in my flesh. In fact, my feelings will often fight me as I activate godly peace. Feelings like dread, anxiety, sorrow, or despair will often present themselves as we move forward in healing. Rather than rely on these feelings to change to determine our peace, we should remind ourselves that God can work His good in us and through us even while we feel these things.

Our feelings and thoughts make up our flesh. The journey to get stronger spiritually is about making this part of us submit to the authority of our spirit and more importantly His spirit in us. When we are saved, the spirit of Christ arises in us. If you have declared Jesus as your savior and accepted His rule over your life, then the spirit of Jesus is alive and active in you. Every attempt of the enemy and our flesh to usurp His rule must bow. However, we have to make those feelings and thoughts bow to Him.

This is where the work is done. I've learned it's not just one-and-done. It's work that has to be done over and over again. Day in and day out, I have to discipline my mind and emotions to bow to the authority of God's spirit in me. I know that every time I feel dread or worry over something in the day, I have to make sure that feeling or thought is not leading me to make a decision or believe a lie that contradicts what I know to be true according to the Bible. Even if those feelings and thoughts remain throughout the day, I have to consistently rehearse God's truth in my mind and persevere past the icky feelings.

In Galatians 6:8–9, the Bible shows us that whatever you plant and nurture will grow. If in times when your mind and emotions are presenting lies, and you begin to meditate on things like fear or disgust, you will see, think, and feel these and their counterparts even more. However, if in these same times, you will instead choose to meditate on God's goodness, His love for you, and His power in your life, God will honor your planting truth. When God honors you, it means that you will experience the peace He offers you. Sometimes, it's not until much later, or even in retrospect, but I can honestly say that I've never felt like God didn't honor my planting His truth in me.

Wherever there is planting and harvesting, there is growth. Valuing growth is a foundational principle of following Jesus and embracing the journey of spiritual fitness. Becoming growth-conscious means you focus on the journey and the lessons learned along the way more than the final destination. Changing your perspective on the journey can determine your actions and groom your habits to be more intentional and less impulsive. Your choices are proactive and less influenced by momentary thoughts and feelings.

Of course, maintaining this perspective on growth takes practice. There will inevitably be times you allow the temporary fog of feelings to influence your actions. But there is always an opportunity to learn from those moments and become better. So much of life has continuously taught me that it's not about being perfect but being perfected. God never ever asks or expects us to do it right all the time, even when we know what right is. All He wants is for us to want Him. That's why His Word says it's in our weakness that His power works best.

Oftentimes, it's in my worst workouts that I have to remind myself of this truth. It's the failed lifts, the missed reps, or the workouts that seem to go on and on and on without me ever experiencing that blissful high of physical victory—it's those times that I know I'm making progress. My body is hitting its head on the ceiling of its limits. Little by little, it's chipping away at whatever had been limiting me and is slowly but surely leveling up.

It's exactly the same in spiritual fitness. It's the late nights of being so desperate for God to move or give you a word that you forgo sleep to stay up and worship instead. It's the moment you whisper a quick prayer instead of a snappy remark to your spouse. It's in the long seasons of feeling like you're going through the motions of doing all the right things and just waiting on God to do what only He can do. All these instances are examples of how pain or pressure in your journey can get you to grow spiritually stronger and therefore experience God's peace.

Patience and perseverance are required in the process.

I tend to be indecisive. Blame it on hosting years of anxiety or blame it on my desire to please God (and everyone else), but for some reason, I tend to struggle to make a decision. My mind chases down every choice to see the possible implications in the near and far future, and I tend to put too much emphasis on my part of the process.

Over the years, I've learned a strategy to become more decisive. In the daily decisions I make in life, the ones that don't bear too much weight on anyone's future, I simply remove my options. I limit myself to one or two options at most, and even then, I try to just commit to something and not allow myself to think about it anymore.

Decisions like what to order at a restaurant or which paint color to paint the walls are choices that would have caused me mental stress. I've learned that these are trivial things that will not really stand in the way of the future God holds for me.

Another strategy is delegating the decision-making to others. When my opinion is warranted, I will consider what I want and think, but for the most part, I've committed to following rather than leading. And this is a hard thing to practice for type A personalities, but sometimes, it's about choosing peace.

As I've learned these things about myself and the way I operate, I've learned the value of being patient. Even when I feel that anxiety post-decision-making, like the choice I've made, was somehow the wrong choice, and I'll have to pay for it, I've learned that God is still faithful. Even when I make my mistakes, God will not. It's this type of godly perspective that will ease anxious thoughts and promote the atmosphere necessary for us to keep pressing on in the journey of life.

> Senseless people learn their lessons the hard way,
> but the wise are teachable. (Proverbs 21:11 TPT)

Becoming teachable brings us back to humility. So much of the wisdom we pursue starts with a choice to be humble. In humility, we acknowledge our weaknesses and sin. Yet we shouldn't get stuck there, or we'll be subject to the pitfalls of self-pity. We must learn to value the process, and to do that, we must cultivate patience and perseverance.

When we practice patience, we are building our faith in God rather than the world. When we practice patience, we're choosing to believe what God says instead of how we feel, or instead of what we see. In my family, we say patience is waiting without whining. Often, I'll remind my children to be patient by asking them to tell me what patience is. When they tell me, they're using their voice, their physical body, to rehearse the value of patience. They have to put effort behind the thought that waiting without whining is something we as parents will require them to practice out of discipline.

God often urges us through scripture to wait on Him. The Bible is filled with references to waiting on the Lord. In my experience, this is hard! I suppose this is why it's such a common commandment in the Bible. God doesn't command us to do things we naturally want to do. He commands us to do things that He knows will be hard and go against our fleshly desires. Cultivating perseverance through the practice of patience is key to developing the character necessary to steward all good things.

In Romans 5:3–5, Paul encourages the church to change their perspective during times when they must wait without whining. He says that this suffering produces perseverance, and perseverance develops our character, which strengthens our hope in God. Later on in the Bible, James echoes what Paul says by reminding us that God promises us a reward, the crown of life, to those who persevere under trial (James 1:12). These scriptures harness the connection between our spiritual disciplines and all other disciplines we seek. If we know the truth, what God says about us and to us in His Word, then we can apply this truth during the toughest times of our life.

In 2 Peter 1:5–10, we're taught that God can differentiate His children by their perspectives. When we see God as bigger than our problems, we put effort into the character God commands of us, like discipline, knowledge, self-control, steadfastness, godliness, brotherly affection, and love. However, when we don't intentionally grow in these qualities, God calls us nearsighted and blind. When we choose to focus on the circumstances right before us, we can't strengthen ourselves in the Lord. We become blind to what God is doing for us in the future as well as what He's already done for us. We become fruitless and useless to His Kingdom.

It's during times when patience and perseverance are necessary that we rely on our disciplines to find motivation. This is why discipline fuels motivation every day of the week. This is why I urge you personally to dive deep into the pages of scripture, and to consider your relationship with God as you continue forward in your journey.

To truly receive and understand the truth, you first have to become aware of God's epic love. Like I've mentioned before, we as humans don't care how much someone else knows until we know how much they care (Theodore Roosevelt). This concept is tested by how we apply God's commands to our daily disciplines. Until you know the depth of God's love, you cannot know or apply His truth. Truth will only be heard to the extent love is expressed. You must get to know the Father and know His love in a personal way before you will ever value the knowledge available in His Word.

**When you're right in the middle of a trial,
this is what you need to know:**

1. (Don't) Give up.
2. (Don't) Quit.

In the same breath, I'd say don't give up, stay on the course, and keep fighting. I'd also suggest giving it all up. What I mean is that I've learned it's through submission to God that I find strength beyond myself. Instead of striving and working in my own capacity, it's when I give up doing and start *seeing* God. You can see more clearly when you're moving in one direction versus when you're moving aimlessly. You can get a better glimpse of how big God is when you stop trying to do everything in your power and rely on His power.

One time, I heard on a podcast that author and speaker Bob Goff practices quitting something on a regular basis. He intentionally quits something. That blew my mind! This also goes against our logical approach to patience and perseverance. The practice of quitting something emphasizes that saying no to one thing opens up an opportunity to say yes to another thing, possibly a better thing.

What can you quit today? What kind of attitudes, behaviors, and tasks can you quit that will free you to do what God wants instead of doing what you think He wants or what you want? This concept can also fit into more practical applications like evaluating which hobbies you might need to quit to make space for priorities. Which items in your home can you purge to simplify space? Which thoughts need to be detoxed to make space in your head to meditate on new, more powerful thoughts?

I'd also underline these concepts by saying that I've found no places in the Bible that say giving up or quitting is innately bad. We have these principles in society that condemn any surrender or any lack of full commitment to things. God wants us to give up and quit things so that we can fully commit to Him. Maybe that means being open enough to quit a job, quit a hobby, and quit something that seems good but may be sneakily stealing time away from God's desires for you. Tune into God's voice on what to start and what to stay steady in, rather than assuming you shouldn't ever quit anything. I'm sure I'm not the only one who has considered it wrong to let go of something. We can be so afraid of letting go, we stay stuck in a job, stuck in stubbornness, or stuck in one bad relationship after another, and ultimately, we're refusing to grow.

What about when it's really, really hard, and it hurts?

Pain is inevitable. You live long enough (past two years old), and you learn that life promises to be hard and dangerous. I think we live in a time where technology and knowledge have allowed for more comforts than at any other time in history. We've conditioned ourselves to avoid pain, and most of the time, it's possible. Yet what I've seen happen in myself and to others around me is that we are personally offended by discomfort. *How dare I have to stop what I'm doing and wipe your butt, child?*

However, I know that deep pain and suffering are very real to many. I'd never want to minimize the pain others feel. Struggles such as loss, abuse, abandonment, etc. are not light discomforts. My heart truly aches on others' behalf. And still, I would emphasize the importance of perseverance and pressing forward through pain.

So how do you know when to stay and when to surrender?

You prioritize the voice of God above all things. The Bible is God's manual to His creation. The manual is about listening to the inventor. The game plan is about defaulting to the coach. God's personal instruction has to be the beginning of all choices—of *all* decisions. We learn to listen to God and learn how he speaks by studying Him, worshiping Him, and reading about Him in the Word. We apply His principles as best we know how and confess our shortcomings, weakness, and sin daily as we humbly declare our will to obey Him.

It's through this humility, this underlying quality of humanity that proves our heart's intention. It doesn't mean we always do the *right* thing. In my experience and attempts, the right thing is not always as simple as we would like to make it. It's not always black and white. God says He judges our hearts, and unless our actions are directly disobeying His commands, then we must yield our heart's intentions and desires to love God so much that it becomes our will to do as He would, to do what would please Him. That may look different for you than for me.

This is why we must come back to God's definition of love. And the only way we understand His love is to both pursue Him and receive Him. The world has redefined love to equal acceptance. The world says to have a standard of love is a rejection of something or someone, and so it must not be love. We have worshiped love instead of God. And in doing so, we have accepted things, behaviors, attitudes, and mindsets that directly oppose God. We have accepted sin.

God is love, and yet He definitely does not accept sin. He is fully just and fully graceful. He is just because He doesn't overlook sin. He deals with it. He pays the consequences for it. And He gracefully extends to us the reward even when we cannot pay the consequences. But someone did. Jesus did.

How can we lose it all and still gain everything?

> If you cling to your life, you will lose it; but if
> you give up your life for me, you will find it.
> (Matthew 10:39)

All my clients come to me because they want to both lose something and gain something. Most want to lose fat and gain muscle. They want to lose cellulite and gain definition. They want to lose negative habits and gain positive habits. They want to lose medications and gain energy.

What most are surprised to learn is that the lose/gain trade-off must happen together, and both require action. You lose fat faster when you gain muscle. You lose the need for medication and gain energy when your body is functioning optimally. You lose negative habits when you gain positive habits. We have to become comfortable with the idea that we will have to lose some things, and we will have to sacrifice some things.

To persevere through pain, we must practice the discipline of patience. We must assess our physical, spiritual, mental, and emotional disciplines regularly. Spiritually, are we losing our lustful desires (food, sex, pride, escape)? Which actions are we taking to support this discipline?

Spiritually, what are we gaining? We must gain God's thoughts as our own and lose the ones that negate His. An example may be that one of my clients decides that despite the way they feel, exercise is good, and because they believe it's good, they're going to do it. There's a belief followed by an action. To take it one level deeper, this client would rehearse why they believe exercise is good. "Exercise gets me stronger, and I have more energy afterward. I like myself more after I'm done working out."

You don't have to know the reasons why you're doing something before you do it. In fact, we perform many of our actions day to day without really knowing why. We've cultivated habits based on repetition, consistency, and routine. We must practice patience with the process and perseverance through suffering as we intentionally work to replace bad habits with good habits. When you add discipline to the reflection/action connection, you will gain insight, you will gain momentum, and you will keep moving forward.

CHAPTER 9

FAITH

What does it mean to have childlike faith?

WHEN I WAS ten years old, I received the "Most Spirited" award on my competitive cheer squad. When I was in high school, I was voted "Most Spirited" in the yearbook. As a senior, I was nominated for homecoming queen and prom queen. In college, I represented the spirit squads as a nominee for homecoming queen in the parade. Throughout my life, others have seen me as positive, upbeat, optimistic, and spirited. I credit any of that to the Holy Spirit planting a deep-rooted faith in me that was apparent to others but maybe less apparent to me. What others would say is faith in me feels merely like a trained response to fear.

Maybe it's a part of my personality to see the glass half full. But I think much of that faith is inherent in children. They learn to lose faith through disappointment and pain. For me, as long as there was someone else to encourage, it tended to be fairly easy for me to maintain a perspective that says, "God can do the impossible, and He can do it for you." What has struck me, however, is that I've fallen into the trap of fear so many times when I've tried to encourage myself.

Thieves of childlike faith appeared to me as disappointment and heartache over seeing pain in my parents' brokenness. I'm sure other common problems like rejection from peers and neglect from parents because there were just too many kids doing too many things also affected my childlike faith. Along the way, I desperately wanted to cling to faith. In doing so, I trained myself to believe in myself more than God. Looking back now, I can see how despite all the major insecurities I had, the only way I knew how to be strong was to be a good enough person that I could rely on myself and maybe prove myself reliable to others. This is a formula for self-focus and, unfortunately, major anxiety.

I would have never known I was an anxious person. I don't think others around me would have labeled me anxious either. There were a handful of times I remember freaking out over things and my mom brushing them off as if they were nothing. In turn, this made me feel even more responsible for dealing with my problems on my own because her apathetic response told me neither she nor anyone else could help me. Experiences like these crafted the lie I would begin to believe throughout my early adulthood—that faith in myself was necessary to be strong.

Anxiety and stress are often products of placing our faith in anyone or anything other than God.

If anxiety had been a considerable childhood diagnosis in the '90s, I probably would have had it. There was a time I got caught cheating on a test in fourth grade. For whatever reason, I didn't know I had a test, which meant I didn't stay up until midnight studying my booty off to ensure I would receive a perfect score. After the teacher left the room with only me in it because I was the last one to finish (I don't know why this was the case), panic flooded my body. I got up and checked someone else's already-turned-in paper. With a sigh of relief, I quickly scribbled in the answers I didn't know and turned my paper in. Later that day, the teacher took me outside the class to ask me if I'd cheated. I'm sure I started bawling before she even finished her question. I was so full of anxiety over not being prepared for the test that the thought of failing it filled me with fear.

In the car on the way home, I confessed to my mom what happened, and the tears began shooting out of my eyes again. She told me it wasn't a big deal and that everyone does that at some point in their life. She may have been right, and I believe her intentions were to lessen my pain, but it made me feel even more unseen, and the anxiety I felt was totally unwarranted. It also made me feel like I should punish myself if she wasn't going to.

Another time I experienced what I now know to be anxious thinking was later in high school, after applying to every scholarship possible. To avoid burdening my parents, I saw it was my job to accrue the funds necessary to attend college. I realized that I had applied and won a scholarship from an organization that I knew nothing about. It also was an award that usually gave money to Catholic students.

The only problem was I was not Catholic. I felt this immediate and immense level of grief like I'd done something terribly wrong. I remember going into my parents' room, telling them what had happened, and my mom casually responding, "Why are you so worried about this? Just take it and say you're Catholic." Her suggestion didn't sound like the right thing to do. As I collapsed on her bed in distress, I remember this sinking feeling in the pit of my stomach, like my body was going to eat itself.

And then another major memory I have about bringing my anxious feelings to my parents was just days before my wedding. I had tried to tan my freckly, fair skin to get that wedding *glow* brides boast about. Instead, I got a bride's worst nightmare—a miserable sunburn! My skin stung. My skin was itchy. My skin was blistered. *What was I thinking? What was I going to do? Could self-tanner cover it up, and would it heal enough in two days for me to not feel like my skin was crawling?*

In a last effort to approach my mom as a child, desperate for her motherly affection, I cried in her bathroom. I asked her what she thought I should do and basically voiced the above thoughts to her. I was craving encouragement. I needed affirmation that all was going to be okay and that I would still be a beautiful bride no matter what. I remember it being way out of her nature to be this aloof. She barely looked up at me from her makeup table and murmured how I was probably going to be like this on the wedding day and that it sucked.

It was as if she was punishing me for growing up and getting married by not being there for me at a time I really needed her to be.

In my mom's defense, she was dealing with her own major issues at all these points. She never intended to deflate me or discourage me. I know that. But these are all memories I have that speak to me when my flesh feels that anxious and fearful fire and that overwhelming sense of dread that says, "You cannot depend on anyone. No one will make you feel better. No one will ever understand you or know what you need."

In the years of dealing with suppressed anxiety and fear (because for years, I still was unaware that this is what I was dealing with), I've found that I tend to be more faithful in group settings but fearful when alone. That's why teammates and schoolmates would label me as spirited. That's why it was so easy to hide even from myself. It's been in the lonely years of marriage and motherhood where my faith has been challenged more than ever.

Depending on others more than God is idolatry.

When I first met my husband, Micah, he was the complete opposite of everyone I had known before. He had to earn everything he had by working, like literally working a job, while most kids I knew were busy studying and doing extracurricular things. Micah studied and played multiple sports, *and* he had a job. He had to pay for his car. He had to pay for his phone. He had to pay for his gas. He had to pay for anything that he wanted to do for fun. He was a responsible adult in my eyes. (He wasn't really, but none of us were.) The thing that stuck out about Micah was that he was dependable. He picked me up and dropped me off if I needed him to. He was on time. He did what he said he would, and he wouldn't tell me something he didn't mean. *That* took some time to get used to!

I never knew it, but I was very vulnerable when I met Micah. I didn't know it then, but I was desperate to depend on someone other than myself. Micah took care of himself, and he made me feel like he could take care of me. Our first year of dating was like a dream. It was the first time a boy was interested in me for more than my four-wheeler and connections to the cheer squad. But more than that, the chemistry was there. Six months later, we were both in love and attached at the hip.

For years, I built a dependency on him that he could never live up to. In addition to relying on him physically, I relied on him emotionally in ways he was not mature enough to even understand. I put so much pressure on him to always be by my side. The fear that I'd be alone again roused me to think we were never supposed to be apart. If he wanted to do something without me, I believed it was because he didn't love me like he said.

I was also fueled by the fear that any relationship that mirrored my parents' was doomed to failure, that for us to be happy, we must always selflessly serve each other and never do anything that didn't put *us* on a pedestal.

But remember, we were only sixteen years old when we started dating. A healthy marriage was not in our near future. Our young relationship became an idol for me. He became the one I wanted to please more than anyone. In turn, I asked something of him that he could never provide. I wanted to protect our relationship and Micah's feelings to guarantee I'd never be neglected, abandoned, or alone again. I thought that if I was good enough for him, he would meet my needs. This was a deep-rooted belief I held for years that caused so much conflict in our relationship. I watched him through a microscope looking for any reason to believe that lie. For as dependable as he was, Micah was equally as nonemotional. Cue the waterfall of *my* emotion.

I'm a deep thinker, meditator, and lover. Micah is a passionate but also simple man. There's nothing wrong with either of those personality types, but let's just say we occasionally clash. For a huge majority of our relationship, I depended on him to meet my emotional needs. Even as I began to grow spiritually, I expected him to grow right alongside me, at the same speed, along the same linear model.

He was not able to meet me where I wanted him to meet me. I became more and more disappointed that he was not there for me in ways I needed somebody. And the more I realized he wasn't there for me, the more I realized how broken and lost I was. I found that through the Holy Spirit, who leads us into all truth, every time I thought I had a bone to pick with Micah, I actually found a bone to pick with myself. Most of our arguments ended with me apologizing to him for some distorted mindset I've been operating in or some lie I've been believing. While this has led me to seek healing and freedom and, ultimately, seek God to meet all my needs, there's also been another hurdle in my way.

Depending on yourself more than God is idolatry.

As I've sought freedom in Christ and learned to trust in Him, the devil has pressed on that original wound. The one of rejection and self-dependence. It's like, "Yay! Hallelujah! I get it that I'm not supposed to depend on others anymore! But wait… I can't depend on myself anymore either?"

That's why what the world glorifies like self-made success and independent singleness is so distracting to what God glorifies. Not only is His glory put on display when we embrace our dependence on Him, but also it teaches us to deny ourselves. If I'm constantly trying to improve myself by my own will, and for my own glory, then I'll never reach fulfillment. If I convince myself that I'm strong enough and good enough to take myself where I want to go, then I also convince myself I don't need God. Ultimately I exchange idolizing the approval of others with idolizing myself.

The truth is that if we're idolizing anyone or anything other than God, we are creating distance between ourselves and the solution to our problems. We are constantly tempted to seek pleasure or *provide* pleasure for someone else, instead of pursuing our heavenly Father. It's His pleasure we should pursue. This is what it means to walk in faith.

In Hebrews 11, a man named Enoch is mentioned in what theologians call the *Hall of Faith*. Very little of Enoch's life is shared other than him being a father and a man who lived for 365 years. The Bible says Enoch walked with God and was spared death, being taken straight to Heaven because he pleased God. In Hebrews 11:6, the verse right after Enoch's faith is mentioned, we are told it's impossible to please God without faith.

Being intimate with God, relying on Him in all things, is how we strengthen our faith and how we please God. This is the goal. We have to identify the areas of our life where we trust ourselves or others more than we trust God. In our journey to get stronger from the inside out, we must consistently train ourselves to apply our faith upward instead of inward or outward.

Faith is most powerful when you put your faith in God. Yes, we can place our faith in the hands of the authorities, in others driving cars, and in the pilots flying planes. There are countless examples of how we operate in faith and never bat an eyelash. We should also trust our spouse and people we grow close to, but we must do so in addition to trusting God first. We shouldn't seek the strength in ourselves or the approval of others above pleasing God. This kind of faith is essential to us walking healed and set free, and it's only found when we put our faith in the Lord Jesus.

CHAPTER 10

JOY

HAPPINESS IS AN emotion. Many things make me happy in life: my kids, my husband, my previous jobs, etc., but while some last longer than others, most of that happiness comes and goes. Happiness ebbs and flows. God put a deep well in our hearts to need more than worldly, emotional happiness. We long for joy.

The Lord says the joy of the Lord is my strength (Nehemiah 8:10). That joy is more than emotional, conditional, or fleeting. It's a permanent choice I make in my mind and soul to align myself with who God wants me to be. I have to believe He loves me and works all things for my good. It's a posture of the heart, a deeper contentment regardless of my circumstances. I may have joy and happiness at the same time. Or I may have joy in my heart and not feel happy.

Changes in the seasons of life have challenged my ability to abide in joy. One of the most remarkable and repetitive tests I take on cultivating joy has been learning how to navigate being a firefighter's wife.

This is how I find joy in marriage.

Every third day, my husband leaves our home and lives at the fire station. Some weeks, he works an overtime shift, which adds to the amount of time he's away from our home. He also has other projects he does on his off-shift days that can involve long days of working away as well. These experiences of being apart from my favorite person on the planet are hard!

Over the years, I've battled the tendency to punish him for being gone. I've also combatted the guilt over punishing him or making him feel bad for working. Other times, I've simply been stooped in despair of feeling discontent over doing life without him. It's in these moments I've been alone and unhappy that I've explored what it means to have the joy of the Lord.

God has taught me that Micah, my husband and partner in marriage, is a blessing to me. He's an addition to my life. I have to learn joy outside the pleasure he brings me. Once again, learning to be God-dependent, rather than others-dependent is an ongoing lesson. I cannot rely on my husband to make me happy, but rather if I want to fully enjoy the blessing he is. I need time to understand how he is an addition to my joy. He is not my joy. He is a blessing by my gracious Lord that brings me loads of happiness. Yet I cannot treat him like he is my source of joy. No one person can be a source of joy but Christ.

This is how I find joy in parenting.

If you're not a parent, and you're tempted to skip this section, I'd understand. But before you do, let me point out that the real joys of parenthood are not often elaborated to those without kids. So there's probably some truth you could stand to read, as I wish I had done before kids if you plan on having them.

The snuggles and hugs and "Mommy, I love you's" are amazing, no doubt. Those bring such joy to me. But if I'm honest, those bring temporary happiness to my role as a mom. The joy I've learned is one cultivated as I recognize my purpose in being a mother to my children and the weight of that purpose. The joy is knowing God specifically chose me to mother my specific children. God delights in the intimacy I've gained with Him as I've called upon Him to help me when I feel ill-equipped, unworthy, or just plain hopeless.

The truest joy I've experienced as a parent comes when I see a glimpse of God's favor on me or my children. This can arise as a piece of spiritual fruit evident in one of my child's behaviors. It could be witnessing my child help his brother learn something new or kiss his boo-boo. It could be seeing the maturity of my child grow as we move from one season to the next. It could be the peace I receive, only from the Holy Spirit, after an epic meltdown among us all, and feelings are hurt, and forgiveness is both given and received. It's seeing Jesus in them; it's seeing Jesus in me while relating to them.

It's been in the longest, most stressful days of motherhood that I've learned my kids are such bundles of emotion and have been given to me to steward for God's kingdom. Once again, they only *add* joy to my life. To be trapped in a mindset that says otherwise is evidence I have believed a lie or convinced myself that my children are supposed to make me happy. I can't really enjoy them if I expect them to make me happy all the time. I can only enjoy them as pure blessings like God says (Psalm 127:3) when I see them as an addition to my deep-rooted, chosen joy.

This is how I find joy in disappointment.

The irony is that I cannot grow in joy until I've experienced disappointment. The disappointment of broken happiness or unmet expectations has led me to question in the deepest parts of my soul, "Why am I not happy right now?"

God beckons us through our struggles to ask those hard questions because he knows if we lean into Him with those doubts and disappointments, we will understand His truth. That He is our joy. And that we grow in our ability to keep our minds made up of joy.

We learn to set our minds to joy like a thermostat—like a faulty thermostat, rather, at first, that keeps misreading. Yet as we practice setting our minds to joy every day, we learn to acclimate to a steady temperature. We can get better and better at holding that climate of joy when we practice it. The best practice is during times when the natural climate is opposing the state in which I wish to be. When my world is chaotic, and I'm experiencing pressure from all ends—in our finances, family, health, schedule, business, and relationships—that's when I get the best practice in setting my spiritual thermostat to joy.

One of the most recent testimonies I can share about maintaining a mindset of joy amid chaos involves the last six months of our lives. My husband and I bought a house to renovate and flip it. This is one of many business ventures we have chosen to experience, and although we thought we were prepared for the challenges of what lay ahead, I'd be lying if I said I hadn't doubted the whole thing more than once.

There were weeks my children and I saw Daddy only a handful of times and for less than hours. There were hard conversations between my sons and me about where Daddy was and why he was gone. There were even harder (and louder) conversations between my husband and me about where he was and why he was gone. There were stuffed feelings and shared feelings. There were long, wakeful nights and early, manic mornings. There were attacks from the enemy set to divide our family and lies that kept us accusing each other. But most of all, there was an intense, intentional decision to find and remain in joy.

In my feelings and thoughts, I felt very empty. I felt lacking in the joy department and unable to meet the demands of being a joyful wife and momma. However, I chose to act like one. I chose to do whatever was in my power to act myself into thinking and feeling better. My husband did the same thing. When we needed to share with each other, we did, and yet we also decided to trust each other—to practice patience and perseverance.

There's a very touchy balancing system in place between discipline and grace, and this can apply in many different areas. In this situation, we both understood that neither of us would ever fully understand the stress under which we each were personally carrying. We had to take our burdens first to God. We've had to learn to let Him handle it and relieve each other from having to carry anything more than we already were. This was a choice to remain at peace and at joy.

I can write this now, about seven months later, that it was all well worth it. The project was not only a financial blessing, but it was also a blessing in my relationship with God. I learned so much about myself and how I related to others through the chaos. Some things we can only learn under pressure.

This is how I find joy in the journey.

Most of the progress we make in this area is made without our knowledge. We think we are barely making it, not hitting our goals, or failing as a mom, wife, or person of Christ, but we don't see the little bits of growth we make every day.

It's like some of my clients who are doing all the right things to discipline themselves in fitness and nutrition. They're working their butts off, and they're still not seeing the progress. They may have felt like they were moving backward. Later, they compare photos of themselves from the first day of training until the last day of training, and only then can they see the difference—the progress.

We see ourselves every day, and we see our worst selves sometimes. We pick out every flaw and every flab and compare our best version of our future or past selves to our worst representation of our present self. That's why it's so important to not only have discipline for our body but also to sustain discipline for our soul.

> For I am confident of this very thing, that He who began a good work in you will perfect it until the day of Christ Jesus. (Philippians 1:6)

To *perfect*, as a verb, is vastly different than to be *perfect*, as an adjective. We can be *perfected*. God perfects. But we can never be perfect, nor should we expect ourselves or others to be. Sometimes, we can ascertain that we may not be able to be perfect, but we can be better. That's a healthy perspective when kept in check. We have to remain joyful even as we travel toward perfection. The moment we lose joy, we lose perspective on the journey.

We have to understand that we will not arrive at perfection on this side of Heaven. God is constantly at work in us and through us so that we are progressively being made new and being made like Christ. The progression of the journey is where it's hardest to remain joyful. Often, we're so eager to move to the next phase or we're grieving we're past the last great moment that we miss the parts in between.

Granted there are moments in the middle that we do survive, just keeping our heads down and hands up, but even then, we can experience joy. Much like peace is independent of our circumstances, joy is independent of our feelings. Peace and joy refer to the status of our spirit, more than our flesh. Even when our minds and bodies are troubled, we can posture our spirit to submit to God, to remember what He promises and find joy. Then that's when we are strengthening ourselves in the Lord.

CHAPTER 11

HOPE

I HATE ASSUMING I know the reasons behind anything, but I'm sure it's safe to say you've read this far because you're seeking something. We all are. We seek peace amid chaos. We seek joy amid disappointment. We seek hope amid despair. We seek an answer to our problems. The truth is that the answer is always some shade of Jesus. Everything we've discussed so far points us to this hope we have in Him.

One thing is for sure though. You will never find the hope you're looking for, the kind that keeps you going after significant loss or brokenness if you don't understand who you are.

Do you understand how precious you are?

If we could actually understand what God thinks of us, I don't think we would question our value. If more people asked God what He thought about them instead of their friends on Facebook, we'd have less self-esteem issues and more acts of valor. It's not wrong to take our pain and our questions to God. If we would seek Him for help instead of the world, we might find the answers we so desperately seek. Part of walking in God's calling and our unique purpose involves us asking God these questions.

- *What does God think of me?*
- *How much does God love me?*
- *What does God do for me?*

I love how John 1:12 reminds us that whoever wants to know God can know God, and in turn, they will know themselves. The Message version says it like this.

> But whoever did want him who believed he was who he claimed and would do what he said, He made to be their true selves, their child-of-God selves. These are the God-begotten.

Like we've learned, a healthy soul starts with self-awareness. Every time we reflect and invite God into that conversation, we grow in knowledge. I'm passionately hoping you begin to see the journey to know yourself involves healing. Although it's sometimes painful, it's absolutely necessary to move forward in knowledge. We then can journey forward with hope in our hearts. As we seek healing, and as we apply the tips from previous pages to numerous areas of our life, we must be sure we fully grasp who we are to God. This truth is what will set the foundation for growth, which will affect how you respond to negative circumstances. This is how we remain hopeful in hopeless situations.

> He predestined and lovingly planned for us to be adopted to Himself as [His own] children through Jesus Christ, in accordance with the kind intention and good pleasure of His will. (Ephesians 1:5)

If you've never accepted Jesus as your Savior, never fully given over control to Him, then I'd urge you to pause and consider how this choice can propel you forward with a peace that passes all understanding. I'd urge you to consider pausing to pray this right now.

> *Dear God,*
>
> *I praise You for loving me. I know in my heart and declare faithfully that You are Lord of the universe. I believe that in Your love for me, you sent Your Son Jesus to die here on earth, to justly take my place to pay for my sins. I admit my sins and acknowledge how they separate me from You, and I don't want that. I repent from my sin, and I choose to give You control of my life. I'm so thankful for Your love and forgiveness. Please help me to heal and forgive others. Help me to know You as I journey forward. Thank You for accepting me into Your family. I love You. In Jesus's name, amen!*

Depending on how deep your relationship with God goes, you might need to start here and camp here for a while. You might need to come back to who God says you are daily, weekly, or monthly. The more I give away (time, energy, etc.), the more I have to refill my mind and spirit with God's reminders of who He is and who I am.

Oftentimes, this is how I start my workouts. I've mentioned before that some of the most pivotal moments in my journey, where I feel God's presence the most, occur during my workouts. Because of this knowledge, I now purposely begin my workouts with worship. I take as long as I need to *warm up* so that I can praise God with music, make confessions, meditate on scripture using my iPhone, and pray unceasingly. My prayers typically begin with acknowledging God and declaring who He is. Examples include the following:

- Abba (Father)
- Healer
- Redeemer

- King of the world
- Savior
- Sovereign Ruler and King
- All-powerful
- All-knowing
- All-present

I might say phrases like "Thank You that You love me so dearly. Thank You for forgiving me. Thank You that You've made me Your child and Your heir and that I'm an overcomer through Your Holy Spirit." This postures me in a state of humility and gratitude. These are things I know from time spent reading the Bible. I'll also rehearse thinking about all the things I'm thankful for and assign God credit.

Then I will also try to think of any sins or offenses I need to admit to God. Of course, God already knows everything I've thought, said, and done, but He desires me to confess it to Him. Making a confession of some kind is usually pretty easy. At the very least, it can be just an admission that I'm imperfect and a sinner. Or that I've been stewing in anger over having to do endless loads of laundry day in and day out. Like I said, it's usually very easy for me to start coming up with a list of reasons why I need forgiveness for the day. Once again, this postures me in a state of humility and opens me up to receive the presence of God. His Holy Spirit is fully invited to speak to me, teach me, and just be with me. And when I've postured myself like this, I can actually feel His presence.

Personally, I use my warm-up time during my workouts to do this because I can put headphones on and listen to worship music, which helps still my mind from distractions. Some days, I'll use this time to go through my prayer list or even do my devotional on my phone. Other times, my schedule may not allow that, but the purpose is to acknowledge God so that He can affirm who I am.

It's imperative we allow God to affirm us before we take our identity questions to the world. Even those we love will fail us when we seek them first. Before I ask my husband to meet my needs, I must ask God. Before I expect to enjoy my kids, I must seek God first. Before I open up social media and check my latest post, I have to receive affirmation from the Father. Otherwise, I will fall into the enemy's trap of offense or a false identity of who I think I am.

Nobody's opinion about me matters more than my own, as far as humans go. I can say all day that I don't care what people think, and for some, that might actually be true. For me, I've learned I tend to change what I think about myself based on the opinions of others. This only makes it that much more important that I go to God first and foremost to get a true, authentic, and everlasting definition of who I am.

Once you're reminded of who you are, you can begin seeking what to do.

Sometimes we have to start moving and start acting, so we can figure out what we need or how we need to grow. This is why I have my clients jump headfirst into new strategies and programs that may overwhelm them at first. As long as I can be sure they understand the process, and that we're on the same page with expectations, I give them way more information and *to-do's* than I actually expect them to fulfill. I don't do this spitefully because I like to see them fail. I do this because I want them to learn through the experience of change, hardship, and yes, failure.

What I've learned from having clients walk through their journey this way, along with reflective exercises, is that they always learn about themselves through the experience. Action paired with reflection will always bring revelation.

Our actions are only as effective as the depth of reflection with which we take them. Are we just moving through the day, going through the motions, and making decisions based on habit, convenience, outside influence, or what's comfortable? Or are we being intentional about making our choices? This is what I hope to teach my clients along the way.

As you learn why you are the way you are, you will be able to heal from your past and move confidently into the change of your future. You will be able to stand firm in who you are today, with the knowledge of God's love for you. And you will store hope up in the process. It's to this hope we cling to as we keep stepping forward into the daily struggles of life.

The healing journey toward a healthier you inspires hope in who you are and who you are becoming.

The journey must begin with knowing God. That's as simple as I can make it. If we spent half as much time trying to know God as we do searching to know ourselves, we might have the love capacity and wisdom to walk confidently in who God, our Creator, intended us to be. Instead of asking ourselves or others (like on socials) who we are, we should be asking God, "Who are You? I want to know You!"

A hope-filled person is inspiring. We want to be around these hopeful people. Inspired means you are moved from the inside out. You're driven by something bigger than you. While motivation is an outside force driving you to change something, inspiration happens whenever you're willing to change something on the inside. Actions like repentance, confession, and humility can result in inspiration.

Motivation works temporarily but inspiration can have lasting momentum. Inspiration is evident when you keep doing the right things and persevering when you're by yourself, while motivation is limited by the amount of motivated people around you. This is why we must have hope!

> This hope [this confident assurance] we have as an anchor of the soul [it cannot slip and it cannot break down under whatever pressure bears upon it]—a safe and steadfast hope that enters within the veil [of the heavenly temple, that most Holy Place in which the very presence of God dwells].
> (Hebrews 6:19)

There are seasons in our life when we are standing alone. In our journey, there will be times when no one else is there to encourage you, motivate you, or inspire you. That's why we have to plant our hope in Jesus, trusting the Word of God to faithfully deliver on His promises. It's this part of the process, when hope blooms from heartache, that not only moves us forward in our journey to get stronger from the inside out but also moves someone else.

Don't give up hope. Keep doing the right things at the right times, and believe that God's grace will cover you when you don't.

CHAPTER 12

THE *FOREVER* PART
OF THE JOURNEY

WHEN I WAS a child, I remember adults asking me what I wanted to be when I grew up. There were times I wanted to be a movie star, a singer, or a rock star. Then there was a season when I wanted to be a talk show host or news anchor. Honestly, no matter how old I was, I was never that child who confidently knew what I wanted to be. I felt like I was always wandering toward whatever I could achieve and praying I'd clearly conclude my destination sooner or later.

Wandering is part of the journey.

When I reflect on how I wandered, I can see that each step was part of my God-planned journey to get me exactly where I am today. I've been a student, a writer, a blogger, an editor, an assistant, a coach, a trainer, an athlete, a wife, and a mom. There are some titles we get because of choice and some we get to claim because God chooses it for us. When I say God chooses it for us, I mean God calls us.

He has plans for each of His children's lives, and they're far better than we could ever imagine. However, He also gives us choices that determine how we fulfill those purposes. The more I've gotten to know God, the more I believe He has my best interest in mind;

the more I try to align my plans with His. While I can look back and see how many of my choices resulted in unfortunate consequences, I can also see how God has redemptively used my poor decisions to redirect me to His plans.

Every time I repent from my sin and humble myself before Him, He so graciously returns me to His favor. Maturity in my relationship with God has given me a perspective I wouldn't have otherwise. I can see how God isn't suddenly calling me to write or to share inspiration through fitness and wellness, or even to raise my children. He's been calling me ever since I was formed in my mother's womb.

> Whether you turn to the right or to the left, your ears will hear a voice behind you, saying, "This is the way; walk in it." (Isaiah 30:21)

God is calling you and will continue to call you all the days of your life.

No matter where you are in your journey, whether you've been seeking God since childhood, or you're staring at this page still unsure about your beliefs, you matter. You are loved and cherished, and there are plans still awaiting you. Your journey won't be complete until we walk through the gates of heaven. In my experience, life never stops unveiling its surprises.

God not only calls each of His children for specific plans that are designed to bring Him glory and do us good, but He also calls us to live our life with intentionality. As believers, we are called to love God with our whole spirit, soul, and strength and also to love people. Understanding the heart of our Creator inspires us to understand our purposes in life.

When I've felt inadequate as a mother, I've had to turn to God and be reminded that He's equipped me for this. When I've felt lost as a wife, I've had to turn to God and be reminded that He's equipped me for this. When I've felt unsure about making any decision that I know will affect my family, I've had to turn to God and be reminded that He's equipped me for this. It's only through God's spirit alive and invited in me that I have any confidence in myself at all.

Where do you go if you're not sure about all this?

While my words do sound very sure, let me be the first to admit that I still doubt God. I still operate in the flesh and find myself outside God's plans. I still have days I want to quit the journey all together. They are much fewer in count than years ago, but they do still occur. My moments of doubt are fleeting, but I still experience them. I say this to affirm those who are still reading and yet still unsure about journeying toward God.

We all begin somewhere. Some of us were raised in Christian homes, with Christian families, and others were not. God accepts us all and desires us all. He personally calls each of us and will wait as long as we're alive to be accepted by us.

> The Lord is not slow to fulfill his promise as some count slowness, but is patient toward you, not wishing that any should perish, but that all should reach repentance. (2 Peter 3:9)

God doesn't give up on you, so don't give up on Him.

When I think of my journey, I like to think of it as a race. Paul compares life to a race in some of his books (Hebrews 12:1, Galatians 5:7, 2 Timothy 4:7). There are seasons where I feel like I'm wandering through the race, walking, briskly walking, or jogging. And then there are seasons I feel like I'm full-on sprinting. I believe God cares less about the speed at which we're running our race and cares more about whether or not we're running the *right* race.

This world is so full of distractions. Our attention is diverted now more than ever. Even on my most focused days, I find myself looking at my phone and being wooed into checking apps, notifications, and stories. To me, these are just momentary distractions. What about the big ones like working at a job you care nothing about, or being in a toxic relationship, or mindlessly consuming life without any understanding of life's purpose? These distractions can keep us diverted for years!

However, I believe God can and will work all things together for our good, as long as we turn back to Him. When we realign ourselves, refocus our compass, and repurpose our journey, God uses those distractions to equip us and project us forward. God has unique purposes for each of us. We don't have to experience one of those superintense *aha* moments to figure out what those purposes are either. (I wish I could tell my younger self that.) We get to discover our purposes as we go.

Your purpose today may be something you define in your current season (e.g., wife, mother, sister, student, teacher, instructor, marathon runner, cyclist, lifter, etc.). And it could also be something regarding your daily life (e.g., to finish this project with joy, to clean this house, to make it to the gym today).

There are short-term purposes and long-term purposes, but they all must point in the same direction as our Christian calling. That's why it's so important to constantly be in God's presence and to constantly be in communication with Him. The more we get to know God, the more we know what He wants from us.

**We are journeying with God as long as
we're heeding His leading.**

When we begin our days with humility, we open our souls to the truth about who we are. We give God the invitation to pump life into our spirits and regenerate our souls. There are active disciplines we take that help us keep stepping forward, and this is how we continue to walk in obedience to God. Every act of obedience is propelling us into the personal plans of our Creator.

Even when we're journeying *with* God and *to* God, we can expect to experience suffering. This is the inevitable and unfortunate reality of our circumstances as humans on this earth. We are born into sin and die in sin, but we get the chance to awaken to an eternally sinless life when we decide to follow Jesus.

God promises us trouble, but He also promises us peace, rest, redemption, and joy. He promises to guide us, restore us, and redirect us. Every painful experience can prompt us to a new perspective of His glorious presence in our life. We have to keep our eyes open and look in His direction. We have to humbly heal from our past and focus our fight forward. It's through these tough times of trouble, we must rely on our disciplines to keep believing in God. When we do what it takes to stay the course, we grow even in the driest of times.

The times I've grown the most in my journey have been the times I experienced the most suffering. Just like in my workouts, it's the hardest ones that make the biggest impact. After I choose to discipline myself and stay faithful, I get the chance to experience the joy of the Lord. Like I get proud of my clients when they succeed despite temptation, God is proud of me! His pleasure with me brings me joy and peace that nourishes my hope for the rest of my journey.

When God calls you, will you know it?

Discerning the voice of God is essential in growing in your calling and fulfilling your potential. We cannot grow unintentionally. We can't expect to hear God if we don't try to listen and obey. Obedience is less about doing the right thing and more about doing the godly thing. The godly thing is less about choice A or choice B and more about your process of choice: reflection, prayer, listening, counseling, and action.

God has a rhythm, and it's our responsibility to get on beat. This is the part of the journey that we determine. And this just so happens to be the part of my passionate plea to all who are reading this to remember why discipline is so important. It's through discipline that we can take action and reflection to grow; we can worship, pray, read the Bible, seek counsel, and then take more action. We do this even when we don't feel like it. Even when we think we've tried, and it's not working. We use the disciplines of our life to carry the momentum of belief. It's this momentum that can get us back on the beat. Even if we've gotten out of step with God, we can get back into rhythm through these steps.

When he moves, we need to move. That's why consistency and discipline are such important values to have in every area of our lives.

We change our direction. God changes our destination.

One of the most crucial revelations about who I am came from this understanding. I cannot change myself like God can. I'm limited, but God is limitless. Even today, I can pick myself apart all day and come up with a thousand different ways I could improve. The world would tell me that none of that matters, and that I'm good enough just as I am. Once again, it's not that God rejects me. In fact, He accepts me like no one else.

But He does want me to change, to continually transform to be more like Him, for His glory and for my good. If I don't give that list of improvements I've made about myself to the only one who can restore the broken, then I'll never journey forward. I'll forever remain in action with zero direction and zero chances of reaching any purposeful destination.

When I decide daily to make God my King, I'm inviting Him to do what only He can do. I've already expressed how I do this day to day, but it can be as simple as waking up and as soon as possible, whispering, "God, I need You today. Help me, Holy Spirit."

That phrase alone, when said from my heart, can beckon the King of the universe to come to my call and equip me to do whatever I need to do for the day. Not only do I now have the power to do things, but now I also have His favor and His pleasure. I've postured myself to receive from Him and ride along to the rhythm of His grace instead of the jerky, manipulative forces of my own doing.

Journeying with Jesus is far better than journeying without Him.

This is how it all fits together. The cycle, the rhythm, the journey I keep referring to—it's your life experience. You, and you alone, get to decide how you spend your days. But you do have an option that you may have never before realized, and that's that your journey doesn't have to be alone. God wants nothing more than to join you, lead you, guide you, and race with you to new insights, experiences, and levels of peace.

The invitation is in your hands. Will you send it?

ABOUT THE AUTHOR

AMBER DOBECKA found Jesus as a little girl but has since fallen in love after finding Him on her knees. As a firefighter's wife and mom of three, God keeps teaching her how to find joy in the struggle and grow stronger through pain. She discovered her passion to inspire others through her ten-plus years of fitness experience as a group exercise instructor, 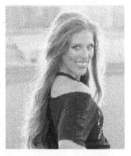 programmer, nationally qualified fitness athlete, and wellness coach. She cheered and graduated from Baylor University—"Sic 'em." She's written articles for wellness publications like Christian Parenting, Forward Movement, International Sports Sciences Association, and local media. After leaving the fitness industry to build her home, Amber continues to find fulfillment in exploring the unlimited faithfulness of the Father and sharing it with others.

Discover more resources and inspiration from Amber at www.amberdobecka.com and connect with her on social media @ AmberDobecka.